Kissi Kurls

Love Your Natural Hair

By
Dinah Kissiedu
www.KissiKurls.com

All Rights Reserved
Copyright © 2014 by Dinah Kissiedu,
Written by Dinah Kissiedu

No part of this book may be reproduced or transmitted in any form or by any means, electronic or mechanical, including photocopying, recording, or by any information storage and retrieval system without permission in writing from the author.

ISBN 978-1494728403

Printed in the United States of America

Contents

Acknowledgments..	5
Chapter One	8
Introduction..	9
Transitioning or Big Chop...................................	16
My Hair Progress Diary.......................................	30
Natural Hair Care..	35
Hair Food..	56
Essential Oils..	60
Hair Recipes...	66
The Good, The Bad & Ugly Ingredients.......................	76
Chapter Two	83
Do You Lye?..	84
Hair Raising Experience....................................	90
No Lye I'm Natural...	95
Mirror Mirror On The Wall	101
Hair Sacrifice...	106
Hair Loss...	109
This Is The Hair...	115
Hair story In pictures...	116
Chapter Three	119
Kinky Curly Coily Tales......................................	120
Natural Hair Gallery...	130
Natural Hair Questionnaire.............................	135

Contents

The N.E.S.S Hair Type System…………………………………..	136
Hair Type, Hype?..	140
Porosity………………………………………………………………..	143
Hair Doctor…………………………………………………………..	146

Chapter Four — 152

Unique…………………………………………………………………	153
Rocking Your Fro On The Go…………………………………	156
Develop Your Inner Beauty…………………………………….	161
Hair Psychology – I'm 'Hair' For You………………………	170

Chapter Five — 176

Interesting Hair Facts……………………………………………	177
African Combs………………………………………………………	188
Interesting Comb Facts…………………………………………	194
Ken & Barbie? How About Ama & Kojo………………….	198

Chapter Six — 205

B.O.B – Black owned Business……………………………….	206
Product Junkie………………………………………………………	218
Hair Diary……………………………………………………………..	221
My Healthy Hair Plan…………………………………………….	223
Salon Directory…………………………………………………….	226

Credits……………………………………………………………………… 238

Acknowledgments

I started writing this book without knowing the form or direction that this book was going to take. Word by word, page by page, chapter by chapter, I moved forward going with the book's natural flow, which is reflective of my nature.

After conducting numerous research interviews; staying up late nights and seeing family and friends eagerly anticipating its arrival... finally is has been born; complete with designs & illustrations.

However, this book would not be what it is without each and every contributor, so I have to thank them all. Firstly, I am eternally thankful to the Most High for my wellbeing, continued protection and for bringing out the creative force within me so that I have been able to produce this book. The universe is wonderful and I am continually grateful for the endless opportunities that it has provided, before, during and after the commencement of my writing.

I want to thank my family, my husband, and loyal friends for their continued support and contribution and I feel very blessed to have you all in my life and for that I am truly grateful.

Many thanks to Santiago for the graphic design, your artwork speaks a thousand words. I would also like to give thanks to Mama D, my editor who has been a pleasure to work with, professional, great communicator, proficient and patient. As you know writing this book has been a labor of love and at first I was reluctant to release this project all in one go. However, after a while I surrendered the pages to you and I'm glad I did.

Thank you to all the models who, I am sure you'll agree, grace the pages of this book and to those people whom took part in interviews ,and were prepared to open up and share with me personal and intimate details about their experiences. I feel very thankful to have met you all and appreciate your permission to share your experiences with others. Lastly, I would like to say a huge thank you to all the people who have been patiently awaiting a copy of this publication to share with their friends and family and who have also been just as genuinely excited about its release as I have. Thank you to everyone who purchases this book. It means a lot to me and I am fully acknowledge what your contribution means in terms of sharing my message with the world.

Mummy and Daddy, I thank you for your guidance and beautiful spirit. I Thank you for being you.

In Loving memory of Sylvia Kissiedu

Chapter One

Introduction

One of my earliest childhood memories which relate to hair is when my sisters and I would take a sweater and place it over our heads. We would walk around the house swinging it from left to right, flipping it forward and backward, pretending that this was our hair, mimicking what we saw on the television. The shampoo and hair care advertisements, and the movies were, and are, notorious for glamorizing European hair and restricting the presence of black women with natural hair on our screens. We are exposed to constant, repetitive images of processed or European hair blowing in the wind, in slow motion for maximum effect. Alternatively, there is the 'popular girl' on the television programs or movie who flips her hair constantly, trying to look cool, seducing the boys, tossing her hair, it would seem, in their faces! To further emphasize this effect, the dolls that I, and many a small, black girl played with, were all white; therefore, they did not resemble me/us. It is no wonder that many black women are wearing European hair because they think, they have been made to think, that this is the epitome of beauty.

Although I had been 'natural' for several years before, I only started wearing my natural hair out in 2008. I felt quite alone in this process. I was not aware of any natural hair groups or forums, nor was I sure of what was out there on offer to best use on natural hair and I did not know how to make homemade natural hair recipes either. More importantly, I knew I would benefit from the support, encouragement and inspiration of like-minded people.

At the age of seventeen, I used a relaxer. At the age of nineteen, I wore a weave. I went natural at the age of twenty-two. When I finally removed the weave and revealed my natural hair to the elements, I kept saying to myself, "why didn't I do this sooner?"

I learned to embrace my natural hair by examining it, playing with it, working with it, and appreciating it. Once I learned to do this, I began to feel more comfortable, more confident and proud. At long last, my outer appearance now reflected what I felt to be the internal part of me. It was a life-changing moment. I began experimenting and concocting my own natural hair care products - that were mainly for personal use. I continued to share hair care tips with friends, family, and admirers.

Your natural hair is your natural beauty, Sistas, I'm here to tell you, you do not need to hide behind a manufactured imitation of European hair, you are beautiful in your natural state; know it, feel it, be it!

Out of a handful of women considering going natural, only a few will take the step to transition. What is it that prevents some black women from embracing their natural hair? The interviews I conducted and the case study within this book reveal some of the shocking, but real, answers.

The mental attitude towards natural hair, regarding it as not being modern or stylish enough, or that the maintenance of natural hair is hard work, or even that natural hair is considered 'bad hair', are some of the excuses I hear as to why women are not wanting to go natural. The efforts some Sistas will go through to hide or manipulate their hair because they feel embarrassed by their natural tresses is troubling and in some cases extremely disturbing.

Listening to some of these women and their stories of rejection of their natural hair makes me feel sad. This provoked in me a response that compelled me to do something to help and support these women by being an example to them; by encouraging them to replace those negative thoughts with more positive thoughts and images and thus to recondition the mindset and attitude towards their natural hair.

I am not a cosmetologist, dermatologist, or trichologist; I'm a qualified counsellor, natural hair transitional adviser, and natural hair enthusiast. Through research, interviews, personal experience, journals and documentaries, I have been able to gather material that has contributed to the development of this book. I want women everywhere to know that having natural hair should be an option for them. This book tackles the psychology and perceptions towards natural hair that enable women to make better choices.

This is where your journey can begin. I'm here to support you, especially when the going gets tough, and the tough gets going, what happens? We keep marching forward, we are not quitters; we are warriors. The beauty of having goals is to learn from the journey so that we can inspire and be models for others.

Natural African hair is unique; people of African descent are the only people on this planet with this hair type. This book looks at proposed explanations for the reason we possess this unique hair.

Sistas, whether you wear your hair natural, relaxed, straight, curly, long, or short it is a deeply personal choice. However, when there is a perception that the hair you were born with is ugly, or shameful, I feel that there are some deep, underlying issues that raise concerns which need to be addressed and corrected.

What you are about to discover in these pages are the humorous, painful and compassionate solutions, practical applications, and tools that will help you monitor your progress. This book aims to address stereotypes and stigmas as well as educate, enlighten, liberate, guide, and support you in achieving naturally beautiful hair long after you have made a decision to go natural. "*Kissi Kurls*, **Love Your Natural Hair**" encourages women to maintain their natural hair, and assists women who have decided to go natural to move successfully from relaxed hair to natural hair. I will celebrate with you on every step of your journey.

There is no amount of Shea butter, No-Poo, Aloe Vera, info from magazines, locks, twist outs or hair exhibitions that can fix a mindset that has mal-adapted views of one's own natural hair. This issue runs so deep that it goes beyond hair. As a qualified counsellor with an interest in natural hair care, I decided to offer my services as a 'Natural Hair Transitional Adviser' to clients who need guidance transitioning from relaxed hair to natural hair. Together we will get you feeling great and find new ways to maintain your hair, allowing you to step out with confidence.

While writing this book, I have had many discussions, interviews, and debates about afro hair with a range of people who work with, or adorned by African hair. This was so as to provide you the raw truth in the pursuit of being 'naturally' happy.

In the last ten years, there have been huge transformations, awakenings, and a rise in consciousness around the world amongst people who have been searching for the truth. We have been under a spell; we have been lied to for long by the media and the 'powers-that-be' about our history, governance, so called 'natural disasters', food industry, education system and financial institutions. The lists seem endless. Within this book,

I discuss the economics of afro hair care and the economic situation of our people, as well as ways in which to strengthen our community. This book does not start and stop with hair as I feel that there are other facets of our society that would benefit from a 'natural' mindset to go along with a more 'natural' environment.

In an attempt to gain control of ourselves, we as people are beginning to take charge. I have seen an increase in black owned businesses flourish; from offering support to home schooling, to producing our own natural hair creams and lotions. It is time for us to rise and for each person to be able to claim an equal distribution of wealth and abundance. We are the change that we seek!

It is essential for us to grow together as one people. That we recognize the importance of building our community by purchasing and making our own products for our own people. This has been the foundation of any successful community, to work together and support one another. The beauty about having natural hair these days is that there is so much more information now, about Afro Hair, sources of which range from articles in the papers, magazines, online websites and blogs, seminars, forums, live demonstrations, e-books, and more, on how to care and maintain your natural hair.

It also needs to be said that we can all learn to respect and embrace the differences that make up the human race. There are beautiful people of all shapes, sizes, colors, and hair textures. In my opinion, the main definition of good hair is healthy hair.

I feel that Sistas can educate themselves on their natural hair; the hair they were born with, without feeling the need to look like everyone else. The Most High didn't create us with the intention that we would all look the same; that's why we are all so different!

The title of this book arises from an experience I had with my hair and it is strongly related to the constant response I receive from people when out and about. Although I searched creatively for other names, I still didn't feel that the titles I came up with felt right.

On one night I was wondering if I would ever find the right title. That night I was going to go to dinner. I was casually dressed, my eyebrows were shaped and my hair was voluminous. I had finger combed my twist –out, creating body and hydrated my hair with **Kissi Kurl**. I was good to go. As soon as I walked into the restaurant members of staff at the entrance said in unison "**I love your hair!**" I thought "That is it! Those words have to be incorporated into the title of the book!" Learning to Love Your Natural Hair is the theme throughout this book. I had learned to Love my hair and by accepting and loving my hair other people will learn to love their hair too.

I have consciously made an effort to repeat those exact words when I see Sistas rocking their natural hair. There's nothing more heartening than to see eyes light up and the corner of the mouth produce a curve upwards in a smile, when a Sista is acknowledged in this way. It's empowering, encouraging and uplifting.

"**I Love Your Natural Hair!**" Is a statement that I want Sistas to resonate with. I want them to feel thrilled when they hear these words and to feel affirmed and acknowledged as beautiful because they carry beautiful hair. What other better way is there to compliment a Sista, than to let her know that she rocks because she is a picture of divine and natural beauty?

Upon reading this book, I ask that you make this pledge: every time you see a Sista with a natural hair style, say "**I Love Your Natural Hair!**" Whether you get a good response or not, remember that when you say or do good deeds and are sincere, the universe will bless you abundantly, this is a universal law.

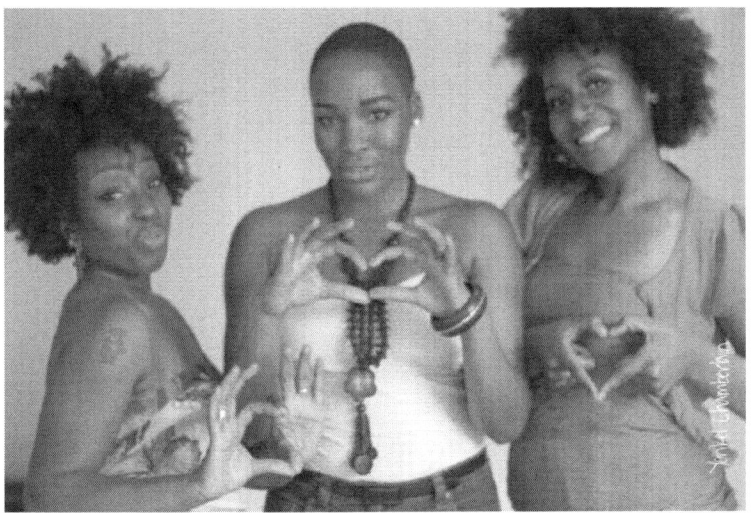

 So, to all my Sistas, "**Love Your Natural Hair**"!

Transition or Big Chop?

Our hair journey is one that is personal to us, you will discover the importance of awareness and change on your hair journey. There is a sense of euphoria when you go natural, I remember thinking to myself when I looked in the mirror, this is all me, no glue, no thread no pieces just me!

On the flip side some sistas may feel vulnerable and exposed and slightly overwhelmed, that's why it's important for newbie naturals to understand that it is a process. Some women may see hair as an accessory others may see it as a security blanket and some feel it's just hair, however you feel about your hair, in order to achieve strong healthy manageable hair you will need time, dedication and care. You will learn to monitor your hair and how it responds to environments, products and styles.

During the previous twelve or so months you may have gathered some magazine clippings. You may have created a scrap book, so that you can try out some of the hair styles once you have reached the end of your transitioning period. Your first year anniversary arrives. The excitement of unraveling your braids, weaves or twist is something to look forward to. This is the hair that you have been suppressing for so long and here it is in all its glory; your natural beauty.

It is a common experience that when Sistas see their natural hair, it's described to be like meeting a familiar stranger. They unravel their hair and can see their natural hair pattern. Perhaps, in their mind's eye, their hair will take the form of a halo of unrecognizably soft and well defined curls. The reality, at first glance might be something quite different! How your hair will look is going to depend upon its natural texture. Whatever hair texture you have, you need to learn to love it, work with it and embrace it.

There's a Sista that comes to mind when I think of 'a nappy in denial'. I attended a hair event and this sista had been natural for about six months, her hair was hair type coily, she asked the host if she sold products that could make her hair wavy. The host took one look at her hair and said, 'hmmm... nope!' The Sista continued to share that when she pulled her hair out that she expected it to have a looser hair pattern, as she wanted her hair to be wavy. She insisted upon having wavy hair, so that she could 'wash and go' and was looking for a product that would achieve this look. The host then pointed to a lady in the audience who had wavy hair type and asked her, "Are you trying to achieve this type of hair?" She responded affirmatively. It became quite clear that this lady was not happy with her natural hair texture and really what she was looking for was something similar to a texturized appearance.

The moral of the story is that tighter hair patterns or looser curls are natural for those individuals who have that natural hair pattern, but if you are trying to achieve a look that gives the appearance of a looser or tighter hair pattern by chemically altering it this look is not 'natural' for you! Even If you undergo a natural hair treatment such as a keratin treatment that loosens the hair pattern temporarily, be prepared to put in the work needed to maintain this look. At the point that you decide to alter your hair texture, you have to be honest with yourself that you are no longer 'natural'.

Love Your Natural Hair

Nappy in denial/Afro Denial
Urban Dictionary

'A psychological affliction wherein patients exhibit self-delusional behavior, believing they have straight flowing, European supermodel type hair -- thereby refusing to accept the coarseness, thickness and/or nappiness of their actual hair.'

Aaron McGruder creator of the Boondocks in **Afro Denial and Ethono-ambiguo Hostility**

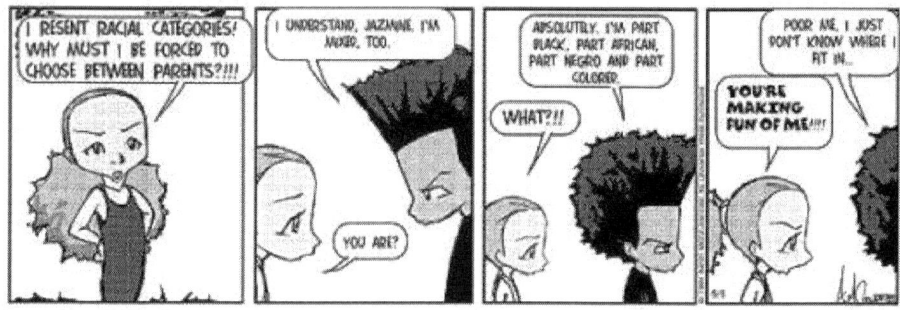

Syndrome

I resent racial Categories. Why must I be forced to choose between two parents?!?!!!
I understand, Jazmine. I'm mixed too.
You are? What?!!
Absolutely. I'm part Black. Part African Amerian. Part Negro and part Colored. Poor me. I just don't know where I fit in.
You're making fun of me!!!

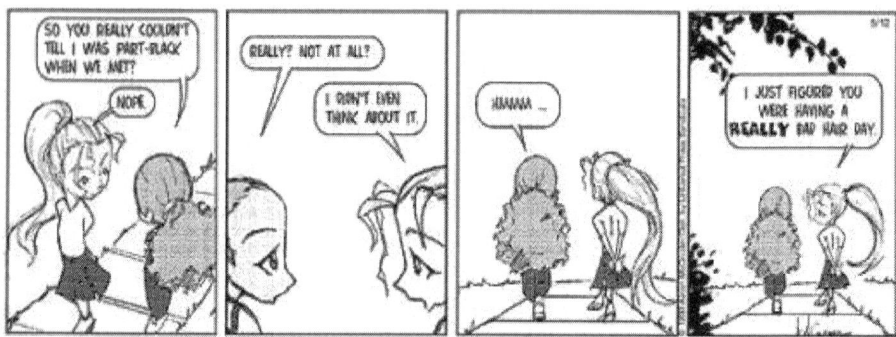

So you really couldn't tell I was part black when we met?
Nope.
Really? Not at all?
I didn't even think about it.
Hmmm...
I just thought you were having a really bad hair day.

Kissi Kurls

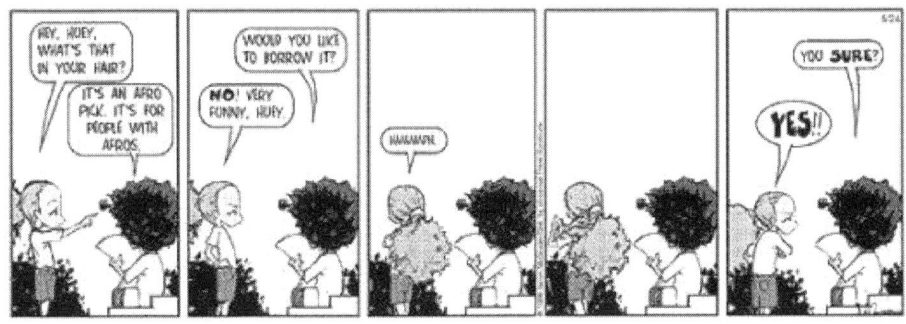

Hey, Huey. What's that in your hair?
It's an afro pick. It's for people with afros.
Would you like to borrow it?
No! Very funny Huey.
Hmmph.
Are you sure?

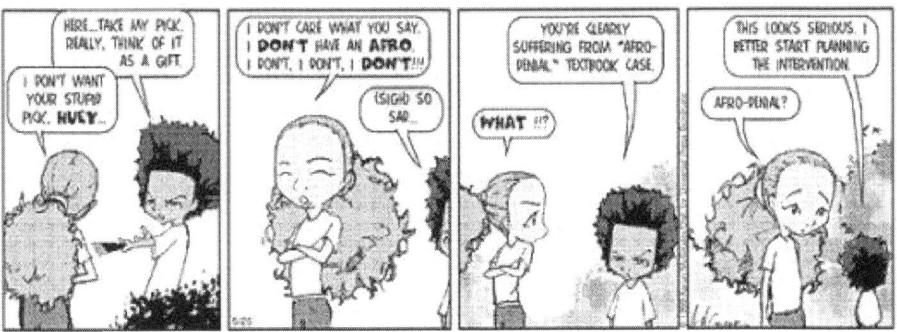

Yes!!
Here... Take my pick. Really. Think of it as a gift.
I don't want your stupid pick Huey... I don't care what you say. I DON'T. I DON'T. I DON'T!!!
(Sigh) So sad.
What?!
You're suffering from "Afro-Denial." Textbook case.
Afro Denial?
This looks serious. I better start planning the intervention.

www.KissiKurls.com

Love Your Natural Hair

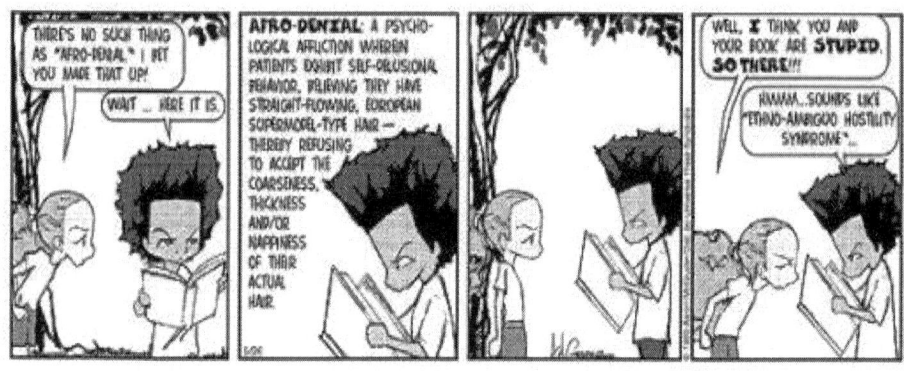

There is no such thing as "Afro Denial." I bet you made that up!
Wait... Here it is.
AFRO DENIAL: A psychological affliction where patients exhibit self-delusional behavior. Believing they have straight-flowing European supermodel-type hair. Thereby refusing to accept the coarseness and/or nappiness of their actual hair.
Well. I think you and your book are STUPID. SO THERE!!!
Hmmmm... Sounds like Ethno-Ambiguo Hositility Syndrome...

Now that you are wearing your natural tresses you will have to learn to educate yourself on how your hair works best for you. Experiment, exercise patience, and determination. Be as creative as your imagination will let you.

The reality for some newbie naturals is that you may have not seen your natural hair texture for several years but you will still need to learn how to maintain and care for it, so that you bring out the best result for your hair, which is optimum health and growth. I can honestly say that natural hair is not 'hard to maintain' which is a statement synonymous with having natural hair. It means learning to work with your natural texture instead of against it. Once you understand your hair, it will become second nature.

The images of natural Sistas are increasing and more and more Sistas are making that step to go natural. Here are some of the reasons I have heard:

- "My hair is damaged from doing a Dominican press, so I have to start again"
- "I want to see what natural hair will look like on me"
- "I am worried about the chemicals and the damage that it's had on my hair"
- "I just want to try something new, not making any kind of statement just want to try something different"
- "I think natural hair is beautiful I have always admired it, but I want to see if it will suit me"
- "I don't know what my hair texture is like and I want to know"
- "My friend has gone natural and she looks amazing so I want to try it too"
- "I am pregnant and pregnant women are not supposed to put chemicals on their head, so I have decided that I will go natural and stay natural even after the baby is born"
- "Mummy, why is my hair not straight like yours?" from that day, I decided that I would stop putting chemicals in my hair and go natural to show my daughter she is beautiful and has beautiful hair"
- "There are many natural women nowadays, and I really like the styles, so I'm going to do a Big chop, and start my hair journey"
- "My boyfriend dated a girl with natural hair,- his ex, and he said that he prefers it, to my weave, I was really hurt by this statement. He said he thought it was my hair. Now he wants me to try and go natural but I'm not ready. I need some advice before I do it. I do not recall my natural hair, so I'm anxious. But my mother's hair is soft so I hope my hair is like my mums."
- "I went natural last week I got my fiancée to cut my hair all off. My hair was on my collar bone and was relaxed. My friend who also has natural hair said that she thinks it may grow longer as the relaxer suppresses the growth and I think she may be right. The girl at work who has the same length

hair as myself said her hair would only grow just past her jaw line when her hair Was relaxed. Now she is natural, her hair is at her shoulders. So I am going to see how this is going to work for me, I just want healthy hair irrespective of the length, I am excited!"
- "After a consultation my Tricholgoist said that the tenderness of my scalp maybe caused my relaxer, and advised me to discontinue relaxing my hair to see if the condition persists."

I have written two, separate hair journeys to provide examples and guidance for the path you may choose to take. Do whatever feels comfortable for you because, at the end of the day, it's your journey and what you learn along your journey is just as important as reaching your goal.

What does transition mean? It means that you have decided to gradually go through the process of becoming natural by cutting the relaxed ends off gradually each month until you are left with natural hair and all the dead ends of the relaxer are no more. I have referred to this within this book as T for Transition.

What does the 'Big Chop' mean? This is when you shave or cut off all your hair, until you are left with a few inches of hair on your head. This is referred to in this book as 'BC': Big Chop.

Essential Hair Care products & Tools you will need on this journey:

- *Shea Butter* – In its raw state normally varies from yellow to beige. The yellow is pure, unrefined (natural) Shea butter has the true healing and moisturizing properties of Shea butter. White shea butter is odorless, in other words it has been "refined" to remove the natural scent and color of natural Shea butter. It is down to preference as to which one you choose.

Kissi Kurls

- *KissiKurls Hydrating Protective Serum* - Excellent for moisturizing & nourishing
- *Essential Oils* - Oil your hair to provide it with essential fatty acids to keep it healthy and strong. Coconut has a lovely shine, it softens and smooth's and its antibacterial and antifungal, excellent for encouraging strong healthy hair add this to your conditioner to and when you steam your hair for maximum effect
- *Natural Hair Shampoos & Conditioner*
- *Black Nylon Tights 40/60 denier* - you can use this as your hair band for you puff. You will only need the leg part of the tights. Cut the tights across the leg and then cut down the leg so it is not too thick for a head band. The head band should be long enough to go round your head and leave some to tuck under the band in case you want to adjust it
- *Satin pillow case /Silk Scarf* - Wrapping hair with a silk or satin head scarf at night or using a satin/silk pillow case is an excellent way to promote healthy hair, as this will prevent the hair from drying out. Applying this technique to your hair regime will encourage strong looking healthier hair
- *Shower Cap/disposal steam caps to soften the hair open the pores and allow products to deep condition the hair*
- *Biotin Vitamin supplement-to help support hair growth*
- *Scissors to cut the relaxed ends off*
- *Soft Bristle boar brush, for your edges wooden comb or Denman brush for detangling*
- *Comb- use a large tooth wooden comb for quick styling (best done on wet hair to prevent damage) also smaller tooth comb for parting the hair.*
- *A spray bottle with water and a few drops of your favorite essential oil, you can use mineral water if you wish*
- *Patience & time*

1st stage 1-3 months

BC - So you have finally done it. You have done the Big Chop, well done! You are a step away from embracing your beautiful curls. Now you have fresh, new hair that will need all your love and care, so that your hair can flourish and look healthy and strong. Your diet and well-being will also have an impact on the condition of your hair.

Feel the texture of your hair; get in the habit of touching your new texture. If you have cut your hair really short it will lay flat on your scalp and in some cases be slightly spiky depending of the texture. Massage your hair for 2-5 minutes twice a week or, as often as you can.

T - Take care at this point as you now have two different textures to your hair. Feel your new growth; familiarize yourself with the natural thickness. Continue to massage your hair for 2-5 minutes, twice a week, or as often as you can. As the re-growth lengthens you may decide to braid, cornrow, twist, or wear curly afro weaves during this time. When opting for extensions or weaves, try and pick hair that looks natural and similar to your natural texture, so that you can familiarize yourself with a natural look. A roller set is also good as the curls add volume and the re-growth will add extra thickness. If you are to braid your hair in any way, ensure that the hair dresser does not put too much strain on the scalp by braiding the hair too tightly. Alternatively, to hide the two different textures at the front of your hair, if you decide not to wear any extensions, you could wear a silk/satin head band to hide the re-growth.

Tip: Massage the head with shea butter, avocado, jojoba, coconut, mustard-seed carrot or olive oil. This will help to stimulate the scalp, which can improve blood flow to the head. This will increase the distribution of nutrients and encourage healing throughout the body. This will help also help to relieve physical and mental fatigue.

2nd stage 3-6 months

BC - You now have some length to your hair. Notice your natural hair pattern. It is not uncommon to have hair of different texture across your head. You may experience some parts of the head have tighter curls while other parts maybe have softer or coarser hair. Different hair type may indicate your natural hair texture, or it could also be hair that has been manipulated by the chemicals in the relaxer you have used. You would only ever really know the answer to this question if you can remember your hair texture before you put the chemicals in. That's why many newbie naturals may carry out a second chop a year later, to see their real, original textured hair. I imagine for some, this original texture hair may have been several years ago or even as far back as childhood!

It is not uncommon for parts of your hair to grow thicker, weaker, or longer than other parts. Unless you want an asymmetrical hair style, this can be easily resolved by cutting the hair so it is all the same length. At this length, depending on how fast your hair grows, you can experiment with different styles: bantu knots, cornrow or just have it out and loose. Accessories too, hair bands, flowers, clips, earrings and so on can be worn decoratively or to keep hair in place.

T - Your re-growth may be feeling like a soft sponge under the relaxed hair. You may have decided to take your hair out from braids/cornrow/weave or wig. Ensure that you steam your hair to allow the nutrients of your conditioner to penetrate the hair shaft leaving your scalp clean, fresh and healthy. At this stage, washing your hair with the two textures may be a challenge. Learn to be patient and assess what the best course of action to take would be.

You may experience a degree of shedding because of the two different textures. You'll know when it's time to cut your hair and get rid of the scraggly, relaxed ends, where you have more re-

Love Your Natural Hair

growth than relaxed hair. So the next course of action is to decide whether you are going to hold onto the dead ends for a few more months or just cut them off. There are no benefits in holding onto the relaxed ends, especially if you are planning to braid, cornrow, weave or put a wig on. However, if you are still attached to the ends and are not ready to let go yet, ensure your hair is well hydrated, moisturized and steam it often.

Relaxer free - Now that you are free from the relaxed hair, styling will be a lot simpler and easier to work with. There are many styles that you can now wear. If you have decided to continue to braid/Cornrow/twist or weave your hair for a year, just be sure not to leave your braids/Cornrow/weave in for longer than 3 months. Always ensure you steam and deep condition in between.

Avoid micro braids, as this size can put strain on the hair causing it to break, especially when pulling the hair up to do ponytails or other up hair-do. Box braids are thick braids ranging from 1 ½ centimeters to 3 centimeters thick. I would recommend braids be no smaller than 1 centimeter thick. If you do not want to braid, cornrow or weave you can do jumbo braids or twists with your natural hair as another option.

You can also switch the styles from cornrows to braids, twists or a wig whatever your preference. Jumbo braids/twists are when you section your hair in larger sections. For variation you can tuck the braid/twist in. Flat twists/cornrows underneath your wig are recommended, as they lay flat. Do ensure you remove the wig at night and replace with a satin scarf.

Tip: To strengthen the hairs ensure that you have a lot of protein in your diet and take a vitamin B complex such as Biotin. You can switch up your hair style throughout the transition from braids, twist, cornrows, weaves or wigs. Or simply start rocking your natural hair after your big chop.

3rd stage 6-9 months

BC - At this stage you may be pleasantly surprised at how fast your hair has grown, or you may be wondering if your hair length is normal for this length of time. The answer to that question is yes. Remember, everybody's hair growth is different and there are many contributing factors such as genetics, medical conditions, age, styling techniques or/and overall hair care. Ensure that you are using your protective styles occasionally, especially if exposed to extreme hot or cold climates. Spraying your hair with *KissiKurls Hydrating Protective Serum* will keep your beautiful curls nourished moisturized and hydrated. You may wish to see which hair products work best for you, however, try not to use too many at any one time. It will take a period of 6 six weeks for effective results. Try and write down in the Product Junkie section of this book the results for the products that you are using, so you can see exactly what the effects are and how your hair responds to each. There are so many styles to choose from, so buy a hair magazine or go on the internet and print out some hairstyles and stick the pictures into categories that you would like to try. For example: wedding hair styles, hair styles for work, or evening hair and casual styles.

T - You may decide that after removing the braids, cornrows, twist, weave, or wigs that you want to experiment with some other natural styles. Ensure that you continue to deep condition your hair to avoid dryness. If you haven't already cut some of the relaxed ends, then it is advisable for you to remove the remainder of these ends before styling your natural hair. Alternatively, you can simply snip a bit at a time until you are ready to start experimenting and styling your natural hair. Start to think of hair styles that you would like to wear and cut pictures out from your favorite magazine and stick them in this book under the relevant category. Choices might be wedding hair styles, work hair styles, evening hair styles, casual, etc. There are so many styles to choose from and you will have to set aside some time to try some of the styles. Continue to spray your hair with *KissiKurls Hydrating Protective Serum*.

4th stage 9-12 months

BC & T - Congratulations on your 1 year, Natural hair journey! Now is the time to cut the dead relaxed ends from your hair, if you still have them. If you haven't done so already, try and ask friends, family or other natural sistas to recommend a natural hair salon in your area. There is a directory of salons also at the end of this book, I recommend a deep conditioning treatment with oils and steam and a professional trim, to keep your hair looking healthy and nourished. You can do the treatment yourself using the steam cap, if you wish.

Now it's that time! Now it's that time to try that hair style that you've been eager to try. Dedicate some time to try out as many hair styles that your creative mind will allow you. Remember, you don't have to comb natural hair often, especially when you have just done a twist out. Most of the styles require only teasing with your fingers. Separating and parting can be done by using a comb. Before styling, always remember to use Kissi Kurls Hydrating Protective Serum, this will allow you to style with ease and will make your hair softer. If you put a lot of other products in your hair such as gel, moose, or holding spray then you may need to wash your hair more regularly, or as often as, once a week. I would recommend that you keep these products to a minimum, so not to have too much product build up which can block your pores; you need a clean scalp for maximum growth.

Wash your hair regularly, you be the judge, by monitoring your hair using the tools provided in this book.

I once met a sista who told me her rule for selecting ingredients was; "If I can't eat it or if it can't go onto my skin, then it's not going on my hair!" Each to their own. Just be mindful and observe how your hair responds to ingredients. There are some common ingredients in hair products which are simply not natural. However, they may be necessary to preserve the mixture of other ingredients, so the product has a longer shelf life.

The beauty of having natural hair is that most of the hair styles possible are ones that you can do at home without having to spend money at the hair salon. However, there are pros and cons to this. When you visit a professional hair salon they are able to advise you, regarding the condition of your hair and scalp. Doing your hair yourself you are not able to see the condition of your scalp and healthy hair is contingent upon having a healthy scalp.

Informing the stylist of how you take care of your hair will help as they may be able to correct any bad habit that maybe detrimental to your hair. Some salons stock quality products that are not available in a local beauty store, retail shop, or chemist. Booking your appointments in advance ensures that you are regularly enjoying a salon visit and not leaving it too long before your hair is treated. Also, some sistas enjoy the social aspect of going to the salon and feeling pampered. Nevertheless, it is true that in some cases sistas leave the salon feeling more stressed than when they went in!

Doing your own hair means that you can comfortably style your hair in the comfort of your own surroundings, taking your time to style your hair and trying out various hair styles. There are many forums and websites that can educate you on how to achieve and maintain your natural hair styles, which is great. However, if you have a problem hair condition, it is advisable to see a doctor in person than to be advised via online forums. I have compiled a list of natural hair salons/stylists which is located towards the back of the book, for your convenience. Use the 'My Hair Progress Diary' contained within this book to monitor the condition of your hair from here on and write down how you feel on your 1 year hair-anniversary!

Well done! The difference between try and triumph is a little umph.

My Hair Progress Diary

Big Chop/Transition Date: _____

What method did/are you going to use to go natural; Big chop or Transition?

_____
_____

Why did you choose that particular method over the other option?

_____
_____
_____
_____
_____
_____
_____
_____

What is my ultimate goal for my hair?

_____
_____
_____
_____
_____
_____
_____
_____

Kissi Kurls

How do I feel about your hair after 3 months of being going natural?

_____
_____
_____
_____
_____
_____
_____
_____
_____

Take a picture of your hair at 3 months?

What have I noticed about my hair during the 3 months?

_____
_____
_____
_____
_____
_____
_____
_____

Other notes

_____
_____
_____
_____
_____
_____
_____
_____

"Obstacles are the things you see when you take your eyes off the goal."

Love Your Natural Hair

How do you feel about your hair after 6 months?

_____
_____
_____
_____
_____
_____
_____
_____

What products are you using for your hair and why?

_____
_____
_____
_____
_____
_____
_____
_____

Take a picture of your hair at 6 months?

Other notes

_____
_____
_____
_____
_____
_____

"If you want to live a happy life, tie it to a goal, not to people or things."

- Albert Einstein

Kissi Kurls

How do you feel about your hair after 9 months?

_____
_____
_____
_____
_____
_____
_____
_____

Who inspires you to focus when things get tough?

_____
_____
_____
_____
_____
_____
_____

Other Notes

_____
_____
_____
_____
_____
_____
_____

"What keeps me going is goals."

- Muhammad Ali

Love Your Natural Hair

How do you feel about your hair after 12 months?

_____
_____
_____
_____
_____
_____
_____
_____

How do you feel about reaching your goal?

_____
_____
_____
_____
_____
_____
_____

Other Notes

_____
_____
_____
_____
_____
_____
_____

"What you get by achieving your goal is not as important as what you become by achieving your goal."

'Remember, I'm possible not Impossible.'

Natural Hair Care

Hair Maintenance

Along my hair journey I have found different ways to create new styles and maintain my hair, through experimentation and education. Along the way I have discovered what works for me and what doesn't, what can be tweaked and what is just weak. The beauty of having natural hair is that some of the styles require little or no brushing at all. The benefit of this is less combing, which reduces breakage and is less stress on the scalp. A 'Twist out' for example, only requires you to tousle out the hair with your fingers and tidy up the edges with a brush or a comb. There are several ways in which to achieve a twist out, and many of the other natural hair styles. The overall appearance will depend on the products used on the hair, the condition of the hair and mastering the techniques.

As Part of my hair regime, when I wake up in the morning or after unraveling my twists, I make a declaration to the universe: "I love my hair!" This helps, especially on the days that my hair decides to do its own thing. Now for those who are not familiar with this practice, start making declarations and positive statements about your hair, trust me this is just part of the conditioning process to embracing your hair. This is one of the important ways that you can practice showing love & care for your hair, unconditionally.

When I started making the declarations it reminded me of the popular notion that talking to your plants helps them to grow. It is said that plants respond to the carbon dioxide produced by human speech, and are able to photosynthesize more as well as graciously giving back oxygen. Although there is no evidence to prove or disprove this, people still take pleasure in talking to their plants. There is evidence however, that plants do respond to sound. In fact, plants react readily to a host of environmental stimuli, as the ability to respond to changing environments is vital to their survival. So my point is that people talk to their plants because they feel it will encourage their plants to grow and in doing so, they feel that they have provided them with a loving environment that will help them to develop and blossom, So, talk to yourself occasionally, say loving things to yourself in order to help facilitate personal growth and create that loving environment that you desire for your own development.

A lot of the issues and concerns that some Sistas experience regarding their natural hair, stem from the root! We are perpetually bombarded with preconceived ideas about what is beautiful. These include images of women with long hair, smooth hair, fly-away hair, dark skinned, light skinned, big 'booty', full lips, the list goes on. Unfortunately, there are some women who get caught up in the trap of trying to fit into the media's ideas of what is beautiful. This creates a never ending battle of comparing oneself to others, and trying vainly to be someone else, when in fact all that is needed is to learn to be comfortable within one's own skin. This emotional rollercoaster can lead to low self esteem, a lack of love and care for self and one's own kind, susceptibility to stigmas, from the media and other sources of misinformation. It's no wonder that some women may feel slightly apprehensive about making a change, as there is so much conflicting information. It's no surprise that when some Sistas think about going natural, it feels like a very big step to take. Attending a Natural Hair Transitioning session will help address these concerns. With some patience, love, care, understanding and experimentation, you will soon feel confident and comfortable within yourself and learn to love yourself and your beautiful curly hair.

I feel it's important to allow people to choose; ultimately our choices in life determine the type of experience we have. I am here to assist you in your journey by providing you with alternatives, so you can decide for yourself. I can help you to take control of your beautiful hair.

By learning to manage and maintain your hair care regime you will be left feeling more comfortable and confident. These maintenance tips will help you to re-educate and understand the various ways in which you can care for your hair, making it possible for you to achieve stronger, healthier hair.

Hair Structure

Healthy looking hair indicates strength, vitality and your emotional status. Your hair not only makes you look attractive and beautiful, but also protects you and helps maintain body temperature.

While hair is growing beneath the epidermis, its outer covering is soft. Once it goes past the epidermis, the outside layer hardens into keratin. Inside the follicle, the hair is growing and is "connected" to blood vessels and nerves. Outside the skin, the hair is essentially dead.

The cuticle is the outer layer which protects the hair shaft. It's made up of layers of protein, called keratin. It houses and protects the cortex and is strong. It is coated with sebum, which gives the hair its shine. The cuticle is made of scale like cells that resemble the shingles on a roof.

The cuticle contains your hair pigment the underneath layer of the cuticle is the cortex.

The cortex gives hair its strength, elasticity, and texture.

Love Your Natural Hair

The Follicle is the pore from which the hair emerges.

The hair Shaft is made of Keratin, a fibrous protein which is made up of three different layers

Three major layers to the hair: From the outside in: cuticle, cortex, and the medulla. The Medulla is the middle of the hair which is a soft keratin layer. Papilla is the root of the hair, the whitish bulb at the end of your hair.

Sebaceous Glad - Produces an oily waxy substance sebum, the hairs own natural oil which coats the cuticle.

Melanin is the pigment in the cortex which gives hair its color.

Growth Stages of the Hair:
Three major growth stages: anagen, catagen, telogen
- Anagen Stage: The active growth phase of the hair follicle.
- Catagen Stage: The transition period between growth and rest. Hair continues to grow, but at a decreasing rate. The root bulb looks elongated from being pushed out of the follicle.
- Telogen: The rest period for the follicle. The current hair is shed and no new growth takes place for a period of time.

Another way to remember these phases are:
- Anagen=Acting
- Catagen=Changing
- Telogen=Tired

Hair acts an insulator; it helps to keep the surface of the skin warm. You may have noticed the hairs on your skin standing up when you're cold. This is how the body tries to keep you warm, by trapping a layer of warm air between the surface of the skin and hair.

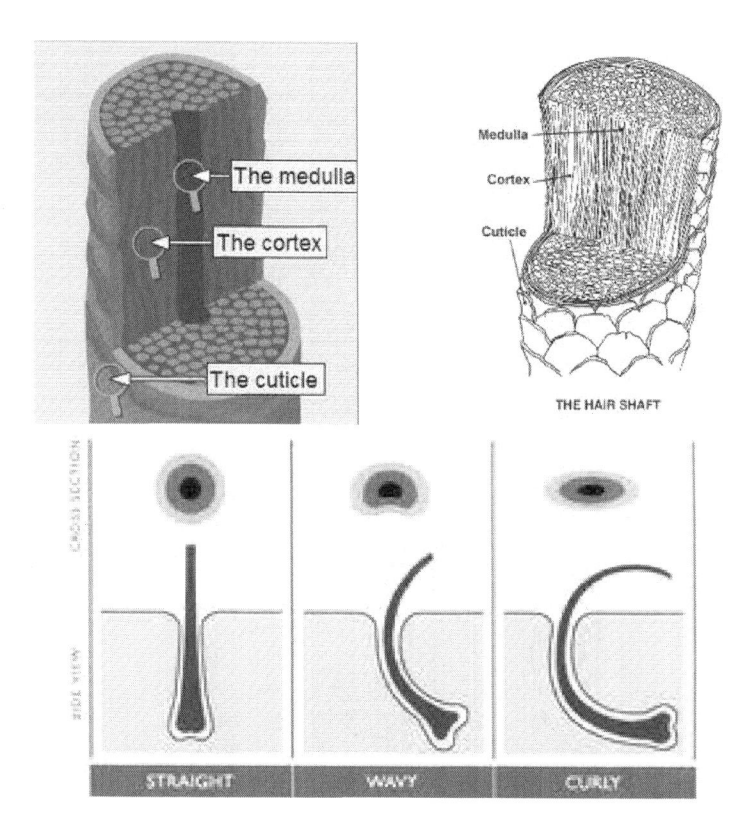

An oval or slit shaped hair follicle produces coiled hair, giving it a unique structure that is more prone to breakage. A round hair follicle produces straight hair.

Products must be used to cater to the uniqueness of black hair for it to grow very long.

Moisture is the amount of moisture water contained in the hair's cortex. It is greater in humid areas, and less in drier areas.

Porosity is the hair's ability to absorb water and chemicals. If porosity is normal, it keeps the hair from absorbing or releasing too much moisture. Overly porous hair cannot hold its moisture;

it is much like a sponge. It easily sucks up moisture, but cannot hold it.

Elasticity is the hair's ability to stretch and return to its normal length. Wet hair should be able to stretch about half of its length without breaking. If your hair's elasticity is low, it will break when stretched.

Relaxed hair will often be over porous, have low elasticity, and have low moisture content. This is the reason why sistas who choose to relax their hair may suffer with drier hair & continued breakage. Afro hair generally tends to be dry and therefore requires extra moisture, and conditioning. The reason for this is that the oil produced by the scalp does not travel down curly/coiled hair as freely as it does with straight hair. So it is vital to use products that have water (aqua) and essential oils. *KissiKurls* products have natural ingredients, and are great for nourishing & hydrating and the prevention of dry hair.

Shampoo

Many shampoos are available on the market today. It is advised that you learn the properties and actions of the shampoo to determine whether or not it will serve the intended purpose. Ensure to read the product label and accompanying literature carefully so you can make an informed decision. The wrong shampoo can leave your hair feeling very dry and strip your hair of its natural oil. The function of a shampoo is to clean the hair by removing the dirt. Try and look for a shampoo that is ph balanced, or one that is specifically for dry hair, shampoos with labels that read, moisturizing or humectants are also good.

Like many myths out there I used to think the more lather the cleaner the hair, no, no, nooo, this is not the case. The ingredient that produces the bubbly lather in a shampoo is an ingredient called sulphate. Sulphates are also powerful degreasers that will literally strip the oil from your hair. They do have on the market sulphate-free shampoos. *Kissi Kurls Moisturizing* Shampoo.

Shampoos for the following types of hair:
- <u>Balanced</u> (Normal) Hair - Plain soapless shampoo is often used for this type of hair.
- <u>Dry Hair</u> – These shampoos often include vegetable oil extracts that help soften, condition hair such as palm oil, almond oil coconut, avocado, and jojoba.
- <u>Greasy</u>- these shampoos will be effective in the removal of sebum from the hair and scalp and may contain additive which help to reduce the activity of the sebaceous glands, which often include egg white and lemon.
- <u>Dandruff</u>- These shampoos may have selenium sulphide (helps to kill the yeast) and zinc pyrithione (antifungal ingredient prevents bacteria and fungus from building up) are often included with these shampoos. Baking soda, Neem leaves or apple cider vinegar can also treat dandruff.

Tip: Search for Sulphate free shampoo, ph balanced, dry hair moisturizing or humectants and see which one works the best for your tresses.

Chelating/Clarifying Shampoos

Clarifying shampoos are designed to remove build up. They are referred to as clarifying shampoos or purifying shampoos and give the hair a squeaky clean finish. If you spend a lot of time in the swimming pool or are in a profession were you are amongst a lot of dust, and dirt then using the clarifying shampoo is recommend to remove grease and dirt. Although this can strip the hair of its natural oils it is recommended that you use this product every 6- 8 weeks or more frequently if you have a lot of build up.

Tip: You may need to use a bit more conditioner or do a deep conditioner, as the clarifying shampoo does not have moisturizers that your regular shampoo may have.

Condition

Using a condition after shampooing is advisable. Climatic and environmental conditions like excessive sunlight, wind, etc are factors which can contribute to dry or damaged hair, which inevitably can cause the hair to break easily. Afro hair has a tendency to feel and look dry and brittle. It is imperative that after shampooing that a conditioner is applied, this is needed as the hair needs to be replenished and protected against breakage.

Instant Conditioners

Conditioners coat the hair and are normally washed out straight away. These brief or instant conditioners contain lanolin, olive oil or Glycerine, to fill cuticle openings so that light reflects off of the hair, causing a shine, making it easier to comb. These ingredients will provide you with temporary shine and may make it easier for you to comb and style your hair. However, the shinny hair is an illusion, as the product is just sitting on top of your hair so it creates the appearance of healthy hair, however the conditioner has added no benefit to the actual condition of your hair.

Tip: If you are in a hurry this conditioner is a quick fix, it's recommended to use this product occasionally.

Deep Conditioners

Deep conditioners penetrate and coat the hair shaft causing the cuticles to lie flat, and enabling it to reflect light. Deep conditioners are intense conditioning treatment that restores moisture, and increases elasticity. The benefit of using a deep conditioner is to strengthen, stimulate, protect and seal in moisture. Unlike the instant conditioner, deep conditioners will provide the hair with longer lasting benefits, such as stronger, healthier hair and will reduce breakage. Try *Kissi Kurls* Silk Deep Conditioner after shampooing for deep conditioning to maintain healthy strong hair.

Tip: to intensify this treatment ensures to sit under a steamer or overnight condition and add an essential oil or other conditioning ingredients so that the hair experiences various nutrients.

No-Pooing/Conditioner Wash Only

Also know as Co-Wash. Some women opt for this to reduce dryness. My advice would be to start your search for a better shampoo, if the one you are using is drying out your hair. The most common issue with co-washing is product build-up on hair. This is because conditioners contain silicones- an agent that gives hair "slip" and shine. Silicones come in 2 forms- water soluble and non-water soluble. It is best to use conditioners with water soluble silicones (or no silicones) because product build up will be reduced. Water soluble silicones wash easily from hair. Non-water soluble silicones do not, they can only be washed off with stronger cleansers that are found in shampoo (i.e. sulphates).

The basic job of a shampoo is to clean the hair and get rid of any dirt, grease and build-up from use of daily products. While you attempt to avoid dryness by not using shampoo, conditioning your hair when it is in need of cleaning will only add further build-up as the conditioner is leaving a further substance, to soften and smooth the hair. My advice is that if you know you have used lots of product during this period and have, been out in dusty, environment use a shampoo. If you wash your hair as frequently as twice a week, and use hardly any product this method on occasions is ok.

Tip: Look out for these ingredients on the bottle of your conditioner, to ensure its co-wash/no -poo friendly. These are the water soluble silicones. Dimethicone Copolyl and PEG Modified Dimethicone

Steam-Hydration

This is excellent for opening up the pores and allowing the conditioner to penetrate the cuticle, nourishing and conditioning the roots leaving your hair soft and healthy. Recommended weekly or as and when you feel the need.

To ensure that your hair isn't prone to breakage or drying out use *KissiKurls* Hydrating Protection serum 2-4 times a week. The hair, like the body needs water and so the occasionally spritz will help keep the hair protected and hydrated.

Tip: you can do a DIY steam at home, buy a plastic cap/use a plastic bag, put your conditioner on your hair, to ensure maximum results tie a band round your head or use a scarf over your cap so no air escapes. You can sit under a dryer, steamer, or you can continue with your everyday task while the cap works it magic. If you wish you can leave the cap on overnight, the longer the better and then rinse with cold water.

Hot Oil Treatments

Hot oil treatments are used to give hair a deep conditioning treatment. These treatments are particularly helpful to prevent damage to hair or to help reduce existing damage. Hot oil treatments are also great for moisturizing dry hair, try different oils and experiment with what oil works best for your hair.

Oiling The Scalp

It seems so natural to me and I'm sure to many other sistas, that once I have washed my hair and dried my hair to reach for the pomade and grease the scalp. However, during my hair journey I have found it is not necessary to use such heavy grease on the scalp, as the hairs oil glands secrete natural oil called sebum. The ends of the hair which is the oldest part of the hair are the driest and in need of more moisture and lubrication than the scalp. If you feel you must oil your scalp, then try using light oil such as, coconut oil or a light moisturizer which is great for penetrating the hair shaft and leaves the hair shinny. Jojoba oil, closely matching the sebum, your hair's natural oil is a great staple in your natural hair care routine. This hair oil can be used to balance oil production at the scalp, aiding overproducing glands that cause oily hair. There are many oils to choose from, massage the oil into the scalp just after you have washed it, as the hair is porous so it will be more absorbent. Oiling the scalp lightly once a week with a head massage can be beneficial as well.

Tip: Concentrate more on the ends of your hair than the scalp, because that is where the oil is needed the most. Afro hair is drying so we still have to ensure that we use oil to lubricate our hair to prevent dry brittle hair that can lead to breakage.

Avoid Combing Dry Hair

Combing dry hair will increase your chances of breakage. Do not attempt to comb dry hair always moisten the hair first with water, *Kissi Kurls* Hydrating Protection serum will help to soften, detangle and moisturize your hair while protecting it from climatic environments. Use this product on knots or for detangling hair. Your hair will appear softer and easier to comb. Make sure you invest in some good quality combs. I wanted to try a wooden comb as Wooden comb are increasing in popularity. During my hair journey I discovered that perhaps it was time to trade in my Plastic combs, for a wooden comb after examining my ancient combs, which I realized had dents on the teeth and extra little plastic balls from the molding process that hadn't been properly filed down. These dents and plastic balls if caught on the hair can cause split ends, leaving you with fragile, and broken hair, and eventually potential hair loss. It is personal choice whether you decide to use a plastic comb or wooden comb just as long as it is good quality.

Love Your Natural Hair

Tip: invest in a good comb with smooth edges and rounded teeth. For overall combing use a large comb. The smaller teeth combs should only be used for your edges and hair around the nape of your neck.

Blow Drying

I like to occasionally blow dry my hair, however, the important thing to remember here is heat! If you are looking to achieve a stretch in the hair then low heat blow drying twice a month is recommended. However, observe the condition of your hair and the frequency in which you choose to blow dry. For those that use the high heat settings to achieve straighter hair note that the heat that some hair dryers give out can vary from 750-1800+ watts! Over exposure to heat can permanently straighten your natural hair pattern, so be aware. The result of this is for example, when you attempt to do a twist out, the curls will not be as defined and will appear limp, with possible split ends. When we blow dry the hair regularly, we are susceptible to dry brittle hair which can lead to the loss of elasticity in the hair. It is important to apply a protective serum to prevent dry brittle hair.

Ceramic hair dryers seem to be flooding the market right now. After many years with the same hair dryer, more like decades, I decided to purchase a ceramic hair dryer, I was due for an upgrade anyway. I was prepared to pay a handsome amount of money as it was an added investment towards the health of my hair. I can honestly say that I noticed a difference straight away. My ends do not have small balls of hair, nor is it frizzy, and doesn't feel so dry. I wanted to find out how these ceramic hairdryers worked. After a bit of research it really came down to the way the air is heated and distributed. A ceramic heater is an advanced type of dryer that allows a more even distribution of heat. This even distribution helps prevent hot spots and hair damage while using the blow dryer to dry or style the hair.

The ceramic heater is also self-regulating, that is, it turns down when the surrounding temperature becomes too hot, because the dryer automatically regulates the temperature, and most of these types do not have multiple temperature controls although they do have a high and low setting.

It is also alleged that ceramic dryers help prevent bacteria formation, which results in a much healthier scalp. Using a ceramic dryer also helps the hair resist the effects of adverse weather conditions (e.g., extreme sunlight, rain, wind, and dust), helps create a radiant texture and surface on one's hair. I can say that I have noticed a difference; it feels like there's more air than heat which reassures me that my hair is not exposed to, too much heat.

If you regularly blow dry your hair, try a ceramic dryer and see if you notice the difference.

If your hair doesn't respond well to blow drying, use a roller set instead. This way the heat is distributed evenly and not concentrated on one section of the hair.

Tip: The cool button on a hair dryer is essential! Once you have finished blow drying your hair, ensure that you use the cool setting button to set your style, and most importantly to seal the cuticles.

Color

I love color, natural colors browns, bronze, honey colors I feel that these warm colors compliment my skin tone. I have never dyed my whole hair and would never do it myself, although I'm more than capable there are just something's that you should leave to the professionals. I would recommend that when choosing a hair color to ensure you consult a professional hairdresser who's specializes in coloring hair. Your colorist should do a patch test ideally 24 hours before to ensure that you do not have an allergic reaction. If you are good to go, then discuss with your colorist what color you are trying to achieve. They will advise you accordingly depending on the condition of your hair as to what type of coloring you should go for example semi permanent, permanent, demi-color or henna. Beware that coloring your hair can change the structure of your hair this usually creates a weaker strand of hair that will loosen the hair pattern.

Permanent color
As it suggests it's permanent, it will not fade, and it makes a permanent change to the structure of the hair. However, when re-growth appears it will need to be re-colored. Permanent hair color, which consists of both peroxide and ammonia, can make hair darker or a few shades lighter, and provides excellent coverage for gray. The color lasts until hair grows out.

Semi- Permanent
Semi permanent hair color is good for first-time dyers or for people who aren't looking to make a drastic change. Semi permanent dye has no ammonia and no developer, so no color is deposited inside the hair shaft. Instead, it coats the hair, which is why it's often referred to as a "stain" or "wash." Semi permanent is good for changing or enhancing tones.

Demi-Permanent
Demi -permanent hair color is good for people who want more of a change but do not want to damage their hair or do anything drastic. It contains no ammonia but does have a small amount of peroxide, which opens the hair cuticle slightly so that some color will sit in it. As demi permanent color opens the cuticle up slightly, there is a chance hair will feel frizzy and dry afterward. As semi permanent only coats the hair strand, any effects it has will wash out quickly.

Henna

Henna has many benefits it is a great conditioner adds strength to hair strands and in some cases, it can be used as an alternative to protein treatments. It does this by bonding to the hair's cuticle it thickens the strands providing strength and volume to the hair.

Henna Is, chemical free natural hair dye. Henna safely covers gray hair, deepening and brightening brown hair and adding a beautiful reddish shine. You can achieve beautiful shades of red through dark brown and black by adjusting your henna with other herbs such as chamomile, indigo, cassia or amla. The earliest potential records of henna use come from Egypt. Mummified bodies have been found with what appears to be henna-dyed hair and hennaed fingers. Henna, a potent natural dye, is derived from the dried, crushed leaves of the Lawsonia inermis shrub. Although the leaves are green, the dye produced ranges from an orange shade to a deep brick red-brown. It is henna which produces the lovely reddish hair color favored by many North African women & Middle Eastern women. It is a very lengthy process in which to color the hair, however there are some great benefits such as thicker hair, It is also used for body ornamentation, to paint designs upon the body, traditionally the palms and soles, for the purposes of beauty and spiritual benefit.

So how will you know if the color is going to suit you?

I came across two fantastic websites that have a virtual make over application. I was so excited to test it out as I had never tried it before. Thanks to technology we don't have to sit and wonder if the styles we select are really going to suit us. I was looking forward to my virtual makeover and it was really easy! Upload a picture of yourself and follow the instructions. Don't worry too much about positioning; as long as you are in the right area it will identify the uploaded picture. Once you have done this, select the style you are looking for and you have an instant makeover! You can use this application with hair colors, hair styles, accessories, and makeup. I tried to find a website that catered specifically for black women, but these are the only two website that I found. As you can see, I uploaded a picture of myself, selected the red hair and was able to see how the color looks.

I would recommend Taaz.com as it had more curly & kinky hair styles, there was not a huge selection but there are a few to choose from. 'Daily Glow' had easy to use tools, however the red afro was the only curly/kinky style available, but they do have a good color range. It is a great tool to use, especially for those indecisive moments. It's fun, give it a go! It will save you lots of time and you can ask your friends or family too for their opinion by sending them a text or email.

Daily Glow:

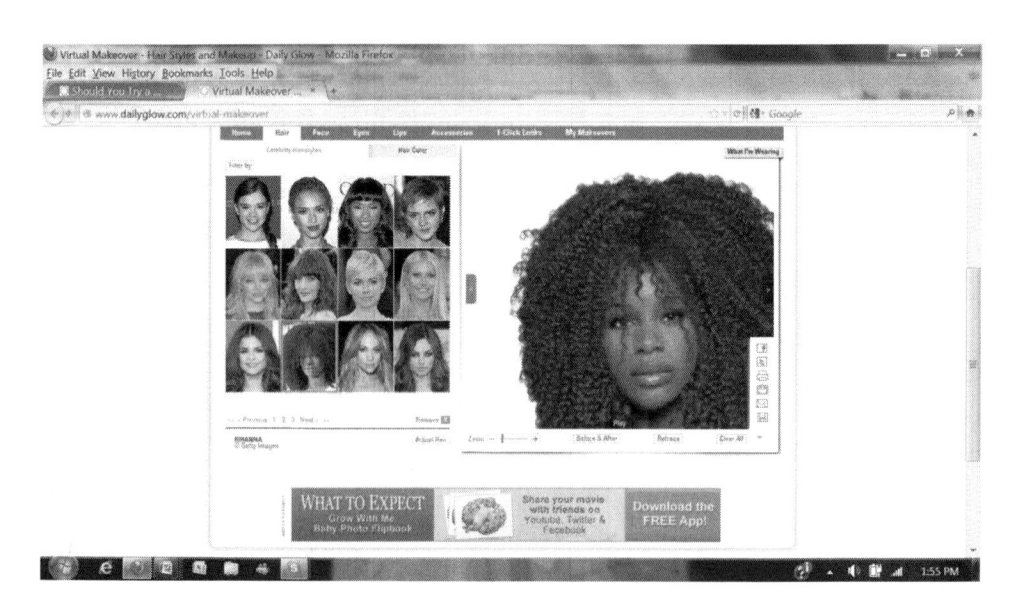

Trim

Split ends, also known as 'trichoptilosis,' there is no true way to remove split ends aside from cutting your hair, but you can take care of your hair and prevent their return. Split ends occur when a strand of hair is split into two or more strands at the end. There is a lot of controversy in the natural hair world about how to trim hair and the frequency. How do I trim it- wet, dry, or pressed out? After much thought, trial and error I have come to this conclusion that the method of trimming depends on your common overall hair style. If the style you wear mostly are twist outs, two strand twists and protective styles such as braids, cornrows, bantu, twists I find the best way to trim the hair, is when you are doing a two strand twist on dry hair. When you do your two strand twist, you will notice the bulk of your hair is the same width, however when you reach the ends of your twists you may notice that the hair is thin, wispy, straggly, ends this is the part of the hair that needs to be removed. However, if you are a person who wears their hair pressed out more often, then it is better to get the hair trimmed via a press out as the hair style requires the hair to be aligned. The frequency in which you do this is dependent on the condition of your hair. I trim my hair accordingly, on average every four months every season. If you are not sure what to do, consult a hair stylist. If they suggest using their method try both on different occasions and then decide which you prefer, the hair dresser should respect your wishes.

If you wear your hair in a shape, for example a round afro, or symmetrical styles, it's advisable to consult a professional so they can shape it up. I feel that trimming or cutting hair when wet is tricky, as the curls tend to spring back up, the length is not apparent unless you stretch the hair, either by threading(banding) or blow drying.

If you do not trim the split ends they will reappear continuing to split further up the hair. Trimming your hair will not make your hair grow longer this is a myth; your hair grows from the root, not the ends. However, your hair will look stronger and healthier. Monitor your hair condition using the resources contained within this book.

Avoid Brushing

The only time that I would recommend that you brush your hair is when it is wet. Avoid brushing the entire hair with a boar brush. The boar brush bristle is very coarse and may be too harsh for some hair afro hair types. You can buy similar brushes with softer bristles. These types of brushes are normally used for smoothing edges.

Knots

If you encounter a knot or when removing your braids, separate the hair width ways before coming out. When the hair is in braids for more than a month it will have accumulated of a lot of dust, dirt and product build up, so the hair maybe slightly matted. It is important to avoid ripping out your hair, so when you remove the braid ensure that you use this technique to avoid breakage. This will make it easier for you to comb your hair.

Tip: Apply a small amount of conditioner directly on the knot, then after, separate with fingers, then use a comb. Using this product will help you to comb with ease. You can also use a conditioner to detangle knots and work your way up to the scalp, this method should make it easier for you to detangle your hair.

Scarf

To protect your hair while you sleep, use a satin or silk scarf which will prevent dryness, damage and breakage. Other materials other than satin or silk will soak up the moisture from your hair and can leave your hair dry, so always ensure you put your satin bonnet underneath your hat or cap. Invest in two or three scarf's so that you are not wearing the same one every night. The grease from the scarf if not changed, will soak into the scarf and then be transferred onto the pillow leaving grease on your pillow and eventually end up on your skin which can later cause pimples. Wash scarf in warm water regularly.

Soft Water

Hard water is one of the major causes of dry, brittle and dull hair. The signs to look out for in hard water areas are: When you wash your hair and it tangles excessively, when you moisturize it, and it still appears dry and brittle, if it doesn't respond to any other hair treatment or conditioners or if your color fades quickly, hard water could be the cause.

Lathering your hair with hard water requires you to use more of your product than you would if you had soft water, this is not economically efficient. With 60% of the United Kingdom being supplied hard water, the North and West of England, generally having softer water, it is important to try and combat this issue if you are experiencing the causes outlined above. In the United States more 85% of Americans have hard water. If you have invested in a water filter/water softener, then you will reap the benefits of soft hair, less breakage, longer lasting products.

Tip: Another alternative If you do not have a water filter you can always buy 2-3 liters of mineral bottled water, to wash your hair instead of the water from your tap. You can boil one bottle of water and mix the other cold bottled water so you have tepid water to wash your hair with. This is an alternative, to the filer system, try this method and record your results and see how your hair responds to the mineral water in comparison to the tap water. Try this for at least two to four months for best results.

Hot or Cold

This method is used on skin, & hair. My aunty always told me to do my final hair rinse with cold water and this is why. Shampoo is helped by warm temperature water, which opens the cuticle of the hair and releases any oils or other substances beneath. Pure water has a pH of 7, and when shampoo has removed the slightly acidic sebum from the hair, the pH on the surface of the scalp is raised. Using cold water as a final rinse can help close the scales of the cuticle, and can help constrict the openings of the sebaceous glands to help moderate sebum production. If you do your final rinse with hot water your hair will be frizzier. People with limp hair sometimes opt for hot final rinse as it gives the appearance of more volume. This principle of using cold as your final rinse is also recommended, when washing your face also.

Stylist

It is important to choose the right hairdresser, ultimately this is the person that is going to help you achieve your desired results, so communication and understanding is key. The ideal stylist will be someone you are comfortable with, and they should be knowledgeable about natural hair, care. Nowadays, because of the huge numbers of black women transitioning to natural hair, hair stylist who may have initially had no interest in natural hair care or didn't know how to approach natural hair, now want some of the action. It's important to ascertain who is in it for the cash, or for the care of their clients.

Speak to friends who may recommend a hairstylist or salon. There are good hairstylists that also work from home so that is also an option. The benefit of this is that you have a dedicated service in comfortable surroundings. Once again it's down to preference.

If the salon has a website, look around, check out the hair gallery, do they say they specialize in natural hair care. Also look for hair reviews online this will give you an overview of what to expect. Everyone experience is different so someone's trash maybe another person's treasure! If it's of interest book an appointment to speak to a manager for a hair consultation. Tell them the history of your hair and what you are looking to achieve. Ideally, a stylist should provide you with a hair plan, if this is not offered ask for one. Customer service goes along way, are they friendly, courteous, and appreciative of your custom? Do they have all the necessary equipment, steamer, ceramic hair dryer, styling rods/straws, natural shampoo, conditioners, etc. Look at the clientele are the majority naturalistas? Check out a few salons before you decide and make a comparison.

Recap: Evaluate what is important to you, Do some research, Pick a salon & schedule a consultation!

Hair Food

This may sound cliché but it's true, you are what you eat! What you choose to eat will have an impact on your performance and general health. You're internal and external appearance can be affected, by what you choose to digest.

Your scalp needs an adequate supply of vitamins and minerals to keep it healthy, stimulate hair follicles, prevent hair loss and encourage hair re-growth. Factors such as medications, diseases, stress, medical treatments, genetics, scalp infections and nutritional deficiencies can cause your hair to fall out and prevent it from re-growing. It is recommend that along with exercise, that you ensure that you have your RDA (recommended daily amount) of vitamins and minerals, by eating fresh fruit and vegetables. If buying fresh food on a regular basis is not realistic with your routine, then you can opt for a dose of supplements instead. This will ensure that you meet your RDA, which in turn will keep you nutritionally balanced. Certain vitamins and minerals can improve the condition of your scalp and help you re-grow & sustain healthy, shiny and strong hair.

Try and keep abreast of the latest news, methods, techniques and recipes, it will take time for you to try them all.

It is tried and tested that repetition helps one to retain information, so I would recommend reading this book regularly for tips advice and guidance. Also, look on the internet for new styles, techniques, invest in hair books, and browse through afro hair care websites go to natural hair meet-ups. Also don't be afraid to educate your hair stylist if he or she is resistant to the information then seek to work with a stylist that is intent on providing up to date hair care, for their clients, the last thing you need is a stubborn hair stylist who is resistant to growing.

Vitamins & Hair
Here is a list of vitamins and minerals that are great to promote healthy re-growth.

Biotin (Vitamin H)
Biotin is necessary for proper fat production, skin health, sugar metabolism and nervous function. One of the early signs of a biotin deficiency in the body is otherwise unexplained hair loss and hair breakage, as well as dry skin and cracked brittle nails. Therefore many people feel that if they get extra biotin logically the result will be healthier hair.

Food Group
Bread, yeast, cheese, egg, avocado, liver, raspberries, cauliflower, cucumber, cabbage, onions.

Vitamin A
Vitamin A is an antioxidant that helps in the production of healthy sebum on the scalp, which helps in keeping the scalp and hair well hydrated. Vitamin A deficiency can result in hair breakage and scalp acne.

Food Group
Carrot, lemon, grapefruit, sweet potatoes, broccoli, apricots, fish liver oil, meat, milk, cheese, eggs, spinach, broccoli, cabbage, and peaches.

Vitamin B5
Vitamin B5, which is pantothenic acid, is found in both plants and animals. Vitamin B5 has been used for a laundry list of medical conditions, including allergies, skin problems, attention deficit disorder, arthritis, heart problems, lung disorders, depression, headache, insomnia, hair loss and a number of other conditions.

Food Group
Meat, vegetables, cereal grains, legumes, eggs and milk.

Vitamin B6
The Vitamin B6 is especially important for hair growth and may cause hair loss when there is a deficiency in the body, according to Holistic Online.

It also helps in creating melanin that gives hair its color. Increasing your intake of certain vitamins, and Vitamin B6 in particular, may actually stimulate hair growth, especially in people who suffer from hair loss or thinning.

Food Group
Yeast, liver, whole grain, cereals, vegetables, organ meats and egg yolk.

Vitamin C
Vitamin C is an essential nutrient for the treatment and prevention of a variety of hair disorders, which can damage your hair and affect normal hair growth. A diet containing significant levels of vitamin C can help combat alopecia, hirsutism or male pattern baldness. The University of Maryland Medical Center recommends consuming 500 to 1,000mg of vitamin C at least two times daily for antioxidant support.

Food Group
Lemon, oranges, guava, spinach, sweet peppers, kiwi, blueberries, sprouts, papaya, kale, peaches, potatoes.

Vitamin E
Vitamin E -is an antioxidant that stimulates the scalp by increasing blood circulation. An increase in blood circulation makes more nutrients available to the hair follicles so they can grow stronger, healthier hair. Vitamin E benefits a variety of conditions, such as

anemia, low immune system, lack of energy, diabetes, shingles and more.

Food Group
Spinach, sunflower seeds, avocados, asparagus, almonds, bell peppers, hazelnuts soybean oil, canola oil, wheat germ oil, corn oil, pine nuts, peanuts, olives, apricots, broccoli, paprika, red chili Powder, basil.

Iron
Iron is a mineral that supports hair re-growth, aids in red blood cell production, helps your scalp heal from damage, transports oxygen and blood to your scalp and prevents anemia, which can increase your risk of hair loss. The recommended daily dosage for iron is 8 mg for men and 18 mg for women.

Food Group
Tuna, firm tofu, liver, cashew nuts, dried prunes, raisin bran cereal, kidney beans, chicken, black-strap molasses, potatoes, baked beans, dates, prune Juice, raw almond.

Zinc
The required amount of zinc will promote cell reproduction, repair of broken tissues and tissue growth. Also, zinc sustains the glands that secrete oil and are attached to your hair follicles. This mineral helps with cell reproduction, hormonal balance, absorption of vitamins and protein synthesis. All of these bodily processes are necessary for hair growth. A sufficient amount of zinc is necessary for hair loss prevention.

Food Group
Brown Rice, Nuts, Peanuts Potatoes Pumpkin, Sunflower, Squash, and Watermelon Seed Whole Grains (Cereals and Breads) Chocolate and Cocoa Powder, chicken, salmon, yogurt, cheese, milk.

Essential Oils

Essential oils are natures anti-dote to wellbeing. Each oil has a specific role in treating or soothing. They can lift us up during challenging times, whether mental, emotional, psychological, or physical. They can help us build up our immune systems, loosen our joints, and enhance our overall ability to be balanced. They can help to purify our bodies of chemical toxins as well as the air we breathe. They connect us with nature. Essential oils should be a staple part of your natural hair care regime, so ensure that you select the oils that will best meet your needs- use regularly to promote growth and strong hair.

Essential oils are extracts from the root, bark, stem, leaves and aromatic portions of the plant. There are several extraction methods in practice like the steam distillation method, cold-pressing method and solvent extraction method to produce essential oils of absolute or concrete kinds. Essential oils are thin oils with strong aromas. They evaporate pretty quickly If applied to the skin undiluted, essential oils, can cause severe irritation or reactions in some individuals. Carrier oils are used to dilute essential oils and other oils prior to application. They carry the essential oil onto the skin. Below are a list of essential oils and carrier oils. I have indicated c for carrier oils.

Vitamin E - Vitamin E oil for hair and scalp: the Vitamin E is absorbed by the scalp and it penetrates deeply enough to reach the hair follicle. The Vitamin E helps in two ways: it prevents the depletion of collagen and reverses the shrinking of the follicle. The Vitamin E then soothes the irritation and stops the inflammation of the skin and the hair follicle triggered by the application of caustic chemicals.

Rosemary oil - Rosemary oil is not only good for hair growth, but also for soothing itchy skin. It increases the blood circulation to the scalp which encourages hair nourishment, and at the same time, helps in fighting dandruff. However, rosemary oil is not recommended for pregnant women as well as for people suffering from hypertension.

Lavender Oil - apart from being an anti- bacterial agent, lavender oil happens to possess several regenerative properties which make it ideal for treating skin and scalp problems such as dandruff, itchiness and hair loss. When used in combination with other essential oils, it is said to produce remarkable results with respect to hair growth.

Jojoba Oil - © is probably one of the most popular and well know oils when it comes to natural hair loss remedies. This oil is similar to the sebum the natural oil that the skin produces. It is popular as it can be easily mixed with any other oil such as coconut oil and can produce amazing results for people suffering from hair loss due to dry or damaged hair. At the same time Jojoba oil itself serves the purpose of being a good a carrier oil in which other essential oils can be mixed. Jojoba oil is often used in combination with rosemary oil in various hair treatment products. The combination of the two oils makes for a very effective hair conditioner.

Basil Oil - This is another essential oil for hair treatment and hair growth. It is especially useful for people having oily hair and when used in conjunction with fenugreek, it improves the blood circulation to the hair tissue, which promotes hair growth. (Do not use if pregnant)

Tea tree Oil, Has antiseptic and anti viral properties, tea tree oil is widely used for treating a number of problems such as flu, warts, cuts and bruises as well as for treating skin and scalp problems. It is very effective in treating dandruff and when used in conjunction with jojoba oil any other carrier oil, it makes for an effective hair loss solution.

Coconut Oil ©-(*Extra Virgin*) light and non greasy, coconut oil can easily be used by all hair types. Coconut oil is one of the few oils that can actually penetrate the hair shaft, and leave the hair with a wonderful shine. There are several types of coconut oil available, but go for the extra virgin. This oil is typically clear in its liquid form and white color that is solid at room temperature Mixes well with essential oils.

Olive Oil (extra virgin) This multipurpose oil is a staple in many naturals hair care regimens. Not only is olive oil great pre poo and hot oil treatment option, extra virgin olive oil works wonders to seal moisture in and can add a kick to your conditioning routine too. If you have finer hair, you may want to use just a small amount in order not weigh the hair down.

Castor Oil (Jamaican Black Castor Oil) A heavier oil great for tighter coils castor oil can be great for sealing moisture into your hair. Many have also used this oil to help regain thickness around thinning hairlines. A little defiantly goes a long way with this oil. Too much can leave your hair weighed down and heavy.

Grape Seed Oil © - This super light and moisturizing hair oil can benefit all types of curls. A natural heat protectant, grape seed oil can actually be used as a thermal agent up to 425 degrees when blow drying or flat ironing. Apply a bit throughout the hair before applying heat to give your hair added shine and protection. This oil works great to strengthen each strand and increase manageability and can also be used to combat dry scalp and dandruff.

Sweet Almond Oil© - This light all purpose oil is great for all hair types and offer many benefits to naturally curly hair. Sweet almond oil works great as a sealant, so apply a small bit on top of your moisturizer to lock in the moisture; it's also great for improving manageability by smoothing the hair shaft.

Avocado Oil © - This super nutrient rich oil is heaven for thick coiled hair. Full of natural goodness like amino acids, mineral and vitamins, avocado oil can help strengthen hair and enhance deep conditioning treatments. You can mix this with your favorite conditioner as a deep conditioner treatment, adding a plastic cap or heat cap for deep penetration. As this oil is a bit heavy and slightly oily its best for thicker or more tightly coiled hair strands.

Amla Oil (Gooseberry Oil) The anti-inflammatory, antioxidant, anti-bacterial and the exfoliating properties present in Indian gooseberry can help a lot in maintaining a healthy scalp and hair. Amla Oil enriches hair growth and pigmentation. It has the ability to penetrate the scalp, strengthens hair at the root When used as a hair treatment, amla is typically applied directly to the scalp. It is great for achieving thick hair, prevents premature graying of hair, dandruff, and increases the strength of hair follicles (and thus preventing hair-fall). Customarily, a small amount of amla oil is applied to the hair after washing.

Argan Oil Is known for its moisturizing properties. Easily absorbed and quite nourishing, this oil is great for your hair, skin, and nails too. It's a great for strengthening the hair. Apply Argan oil for a natural, flexible, long lasting hold. Without stiffness or stickiness your style will stay in place all day long.

Rose Oil: A light weight oil, rose oil is perfect for waves or those with thinner hair. Rose oil strengthens hair at the root and protects against frizz and adds shine.

Chamomile Oil: chamomile is known to soothe the nerves and it does the same for your hair and scalp, in fact it is the most soothing of the essential oils for the hair and scalp. Chamomile helps to retract skin cells that have been inflamed from chemical procedures and harsh weather conditions and helps with itching scaly scalp and dandruff.

Peppermint Oil: helps to stimulate blood flow to the root of the hair. This is very important for hair, as it helps the hair to receive proper nourishment. This in turn will lead to hair growth. That tingly feeling when peppermint oil is felt on the scalp is actually the stimulation of blood flow to hair.

Lemon Oil: is especially beneficial for oily hair, it is recommended that persons with dry hair not use lemon oil, it is a good treatment for dry scalp, dandruff, lice, and under-active sebaceous glands.

Myrrh Oil: myrrh is very good for dry hair. It helps with the treatment for dry scalp, dandruff problems and under-active sebaceous glands. Use instead of lemon oil if your hair is not oily.

Burdock Oil
Burdock essential oil is good for the scalp and encourages hair growth. It is also good for the skin, scalp and hair cell renewal, and stimulates blood flow to the root of the hair. It helps with the problem of hair loss.

Ylang Ylang Oil

Like Lavender, it is thought to reduce stress. Long used to increase the thickness of the hair shaft and to grow thicker hair. Can have a balancing effect on scalp oil production, and may help with split ends.

Making your own natural hair conditioner is a great way to target hair treatments to your specific hair type - without unhealthy chemicals or synthetic additives. The best oils for your hair type:

<u>Normal Hair</u>
Thyme oil, sage oil, Jojoba Oil, Olive Oil, Virgin Coconut Oil

<u>Dry, Damaged or Frizzy Hair</u>
Castor Oil, Jojoba Oil, Olive Oil, Shea Butter, Virgin Coconut Oil, Lavender, Geranium, Myrrh Oil

<u>Oily Hair</u>
Grapeseed Oil, Jojoba Oil, cedar wood, cypress oil, Eucalyptus oil, Lemon Oil

<u>Thinning Hair</u>
Avocado Oil, Amla Oil, Castor Oil, Grapeseed Oil, Olive Oil, Sweet Almond Oil

<u>Dandruff</u>
Avocado Oil, Amla Oil, Castor Oil, Olive Oil, Sesame Oil, Virgin Coconut Oil

Hair Recipes

The beauty of making your own recipes is most of the products you probably already have in the kitchen. All the ingredients needed are natural and cost effective. I must admit I don't routinely measure my ingredients; I just go with the flow. I check the condition of my hair this works best for me. Below are some of my natural home hair recipes, that work wonders, and recipes from other naturals in the natural hair care world. The results will vary depending on hair texture and condition and length of time the product is left on the hair. Try making your own concoctions and see what recipes work for you.

Soothing Hair Moisturizer spray
Ingredients:
- 4/5 oz/ 115ml bottle
- Glycerin
- Water(bottled spring water is good)
- 20 drops Lavender Oil
- 3 tbs Coconut oil

For easy quick everyday moisturizing and hydrating you can use this hair soothing moisture recipe which is quick and easy. Fill the bottle half way with water. Then fill the bottle 30% of the way with glycerin. Add 20 drops of lavender oil, and 3 tbsp of coconut oil and shake well. Spray the hair at a distance before styling and detangling. This soothing moisturizing spray is great because the lavender has a calming effect and acts as an anti-bacterial agent. This soothing hair moisturizing spray also possess several regenerative properties which make it ideal for treating skin and scalp problems such as dandruff, itchiness and hair loss.

The coconut oil adds shine and it is an excellent conditioner and helps in the re-growth of damaged hair. It also provides the essential proteins required for nourishing damaged hair. The water hydrates and the glycerin softens and moisturizes.

Deep conditioning Treatment
Ingredients:
- Deep Conditioner
- 2tbs Jojoba oil
- 2tbs Coconut Oil
- Conditioner
- Heat Cap
- 1 container
- Mixing bowl
- 1 Egg
- Spoon

Place the conditioner of your choice into a bowl, mix in all the ingredients with a spoon or your hand and apply conditioner from root to tip on your hair. Cover your hair with the steam cap for 30 minutes. The longer you leave it the better. Remove the cap and wash with cold water. Do not wash with hot water otherwise you could have scrambled egg on your head!

Rich Protein Conditioner
Ingredients:
- 2 eggs
- Handful of Okra
- Conditioner

Blend three ingredients apply to the hair. Put a heat cap on for 30 minutes, rinse in cold water. Your hair will feel soft and look great.

Ingredients:
- 1 Egg
- 2 tablespoons of Coconut oil
- ½ Avocados

Beat egg and oil and then add the avocado and mix well until creamy. Distribute throughout hair and leave on for 20 minutes and rinse thoroughly with tepid water.

Tea Rinse
Ingredients:
- Tea/black/green/white
- Spray bottle

Tea rinse is done by pouring a cup of tea, commonly green or black, over the hair to reduce shedding or stimulate hair growth. The caffeine in the tea penetrates the hair follicles. Black tea has more caffeine therefore will not need to sit for as long as the green or white tea. Pour hot water over tea bag. Allow to sit for 1-2 minutes remove tea bag and allow cooling to lukewarm. Pour tea in spray bottle and spray the entire head. Leave on between 5-30 minutes, then shampoo and conditioner as usual.

Creamy Fluffy Shea Butter
Ingredients:
- Unrefined Shea Butter
- 1 tbs coconut Oil
- 1 tbs Jojoba Oil
- 1 tsp Castor Oil
- ½ tsp Vit E Oil
- 1 tsp Olive Oil
- Blender
- Container

- Spoon knife
- Plastic bag

Mix ingredients in a bowl until fluffy. Using the spoon, scoop up the contents into the plastic bag. Pierce a hole in the corner of the bag (like an icing bag) and squeeze the fluffy Shea butter into the container.

Flax seed Gel

Ingredients:
- Vit E
- Basil
- Rosemary
- Ylang Ylang
- Lavendar
- Pantyhose
- ¼ cup flax seed
- 2 cups of water
- Tongs
- container

Pour flax seed into saucepan and 2 cups of water and mix and stir occasionally so the seeds do not stick to the bottom of the pan. The water will thicken and congeal and the mucous will float to the top of the pan. The water will become thick. Bring to a boil and pour contents into panty hose, over the container. Use the tongs to squeeze the liquid from the flax seed into a container and add essential oils and mix. Source: Naptural85

Avocado Deep Hair Conditioner

Ingredients:
- 1 small jar of mayonnaise
- 1/2 avocado

Peel avocado and remove pit. Mix all ingredients in a medium-sized bowl with your hands until it's a consistent green color. Smooth into hair being careful to work it to the ends. Use shower cap or plastic wrap to seal body heat in. Leave on hair for 30 minutes. For deeper conditioning wrap a hot, damp towel around your head over the plastic, or use a hair dryer set to a low to medium heat setting.

Ginger Dandruff Treatment

Ingredients:
- Ginger root
- 1 teaspoon organic sesame oil
- 1 teaspoon lemon juice

Squeeze ginger root through press to obtain one tablespoon of juice. Mix all ingredients. Apply to scalp and let dry before shampooing. Repeat three times a week. Source: Longlocks

Clarifying Shampoo

Ingredients:
- 2 cups of water
- ½ Lemon

This natural clarifying treatment will remove build up. Mix ingredients together and allow to sit on the hair for fifteen minutes. Rinse and condition the hair with cold water and style as desired.

Chamomile Fields Shampoo

Ingredients:
- 4 bags of Chamomile tea (or 1 handful of fresh Chamomile flowers)
- 4 tablespoons pure soap flakes
- 1 1/2 tablespoons glycerin*

Let the tea bags steep in 1 1/2 cups of boiled water for 10 minutes. Remove the tea bags and with the remaining liquid add the soap flakes. Let stand until the soap softens. Stir in glycerin until mixture is well blended. Pour into a bottle. Keep in a dark, cool place. Source: Pioneer Thinking

Olive Oil Hair Mask

Ingredients:
- Honey
- Olive Oil

Combine 2 tablespoon honey and 3 tablespoon olive oil together. Apply thoroughly and then cover with plastic wrap and set for 15 minutes.

Apple Cider Vinegar Rinse

Ingredients:
- Cup Of Apple Cider Vinegar
- 2 cups of water

Mix together and distribute throughout the hair evenly leave on for 2-3 minutes. Use as a final rinse after shampooing and rinsing with cold water.

Scalp Energizer

Ingredients:
- 2 drops pure peppermint Oil
- 4oz Water
- Spray Bottle

Pour ingredients into spray bottle shake and apply to scalp. Refreshing scalp energizer.

Love Your Natural Hair

Brown Sugar Scalp scrub

Ingredients:
- 1 ½ tbs brown sugar
- 3 tbs conditioner
- 2tbsOlive Oil
- 3tbs Lavender

Mix together and apply to scalp and massage gently. Rinse then shampoo. Finish with a cold rinse. Great tension release treatment.

Dry Hair- Shampoo

Ingredients:
- ½ Water
- ¼ Castile Soap
- ½ tsp Jojoba dry hair /grape seed Oil for oily hair

Mix all of the ingredients together and pour into a clean squeeze bottle. Let mixture thicken overnight, and then use just like any other shampoo. Final rinse with cool water.

Baking Soda Clarifier for Heavy Hair Product Build-Up

Ingredients:
- 3 tablespoons baking soda
- 1 1/2 teaspoons creamy honey
- 1/4 teaspoon water
- Cider Vinegar Clarifying Hair Rinse

Mix ingredients together to form a paste. Add additional water, a few drops at a time, if the mixture is too thick. Shampoo hair as usual. Apply mixture to hair and leave on for up to five minutes. Rinse hair as usual. Poor Cider Vinegar Clarifying Rinse through hair, do not rinse again [the cider vinegar scent will very quickly dissipate]. If your hair is "squeaky clean" apply a light, silicone-free conditioner or silicone-free leave-in conditioner. This is best used for first-time clarifying, by those who use a full line of hair products that include silicone that have left behind a heavy build-up, or those who clarify rarely.

Remedies For Thicker Hair

Ingredients:
- ½ Avocado
- 2 tbsp Olive oil

Add two tablespoons of olive oil to half a ripe mashed avocado. Apply this hair mask on freshly shampooed hair and allow it to sit for about thirty minutes. Finally rinse your hair thoroughly and apply some conditioner.

Ingredients:
- Aloe Vera
- 1 Egg

Extract the gel from one or two Aloe Vera leaves and rub the gel onto the scalp and allow it to sit for half an hour before rinsing your hair with lukewarm water. Another option is to mix the Aloe Vera gel with one egg. Apply this mixture to your scalp and after ten to fifteen minutes shampoo your hair. Follow this remedy once a week to enjoy thicker and healthy hair. At the same time you can also consume one tablespoon of Aloe Vera juice daily on an empty stomach to enjoy better hair growth.

Ingredients:
- 3 Tablespoons Amla Oil
- 1 Egg

Beat the egg and amla oil in a bowl and distribute throughout hair from scalp to ends of the hair. For deep conditioning hair can be covered with a shower cap. After sitting for 15 minutes or more, rinse thoroughly from the hair with tepid water, do not use hot water when you have egg as an ingredient otherwise you will have scrambled hair on your head!

Deep Conditioning Treatment
Ingredients:
- A bowl
- An avocado (I used half)
- 2 tbs of olive oil
- 2 tbs spoons of honey

Put this in after your wash session and cover with a shower cap. Leave in for 30 minutes to an hour. Source: Loveandafro

Hot Oil Treatment for Damaged Hair
Ingredients:
- 1/2 cup organic soybean oil or organic sunflower oil
- 8 drops oil of sandalwood
- 8 drops oil of lavender
- 8 drops oil of geranium

Mix all ingredients well. Warm oil to a comfortable temperature and apply the mixture to damp hair. Wrap hair in plastic wrap and apply a hot towel for 20 minutes and then Shampoo.

Herbs for Hair
Herbs can also be used to help treat the hair. The herbs mentioned can be used for specific conditions try adding some of the herbs to your hair regime:

Normal hair: Basil, Calendula, Chamomile, Horsetail, Lavender, Linden flowers, Nettle, Parsley leaf, Rosemary, Sage, Watercress

Dry hair and scalp: Burdock root, Calendula, Chamomile, Comfrey leaf, Elder flowers, Horsetail, Lavender, Marshmallow root, Nettle, Parsley leaf, Sage.

Oily hair and scalp: Bay leaf, Burdock root, Calendula, Chamomile, Horsetail, Lemon Balm, Lavender, Lemon peel, Lemongrass, Nettle, Peppermint, Rosemary, Thyme, Witch Hazel bark, Yarrow leaf and flower.

Scalp conditions (dandruff, sensitive skin, inflammation, itchiness, dermatitis): Burdock root, Calendula, Chamomile, Comfrey leaf, Eucalyptus, Horsetail, Lavender, Marshmallow root, Nettle, Oregano, Peppermint, Rosemary, Sage, Thyme.

Hair loss/thinning: Basil, Nettle, Rosemary, Sage.

Golden highlights: Calendula, Chamomile, Lemon, Sunflower petals.

Dark highlights: Black Tea, Black Walnut hulls (crushed or chopped), Comfrey root, Nettle, Rosemary, Sage.

Red highlights: Calendula, Henna, Hibiscus flowers, Red Clover flowers, Rose hips, Red Rose petals. Source: herbfest

The Good, The Bad & Ugly - Ingredients

Sodium-me-thing-am-a-jigi ?

The amount of letters used for some of the ingredients in hair products can be daunting, it is a task just to pronounce some of these words, especially where it feels like they have used all the letters in the alphabet just to confuse and distract you, preventing you from knowing what these ingredients mean and do.

So how important is it to know what these ingredients are and do?

Just like food ingredients, where some people have an aversion to nuts, milk, pork, or other foods that can play havoc with one's health, it's also just as important to know what ingredients you put on your skin, so that you are not exposing yourself to an ingredient that could be doing you more bad than good. It is very easy to get caught up in the slogans that promise long, healthy hair with pretty packaging, highlighting that the product is 'natural'. However, as I have found, some of the brands can be misleading and further investigation may reveal that many of the ingredients are synthetic, including harsh chemicals that can be harmful, stripping your hair or making it feel heavy, dry and brittle. I know that reading the labels might seem like a bore - and you may have to squint - reading the ingredients on some of these packages, as the writing is so small! However, if your aim is to be aware of what these ingredients are and how they can affect you, then it's necessary, so you can make a wise purchase decision.

Below is a brief outline of some the ingredients that may potentially cause cancer (carcinogenic) and hormone altering chemicals.

The Bad...

Propylene Glycol, (PPG) is an anti freeze, that is used for your car radiator, hand sanitizers, moisturizers, shaving creams, deodorants, mouth wash and baby products. Propylene Glycol is an organic alcohol. It is one of the most widely used ingredients in cosmetics and personal care products. It has been known to cause allergic reactions, hives, dermatitis, dry skin and eczema.

Parabens (butylparabean, methylparaben, ethylparaben are the most widely used group of preservatives in cosmetics. It is estimated that 90% of all cosmetics products contain parabens. Recent studies have shown that parabens have been found in human breast tumors.

Sodium Lauryl/Laureth Sulphate (SLS)
SLS is used primarily as a detergent cleanser and can strip the hair of its natural oils, often leaving it dry and brittle. Evidence has shown it is a skin irritant however it is not toxic or dangerous instead it may cause allergic or sensitizing reactions for many people.

Diethanolamine (DEA) Triehanolamine (TEA)
Diethanolamine is a colorless liquid used as a ph adjuster, also used as a lather agent. DEA is used widely because it provides a rich lather in shampoos and keeps a favorable consistency in lotions and creams. DEA can react with other ingredients in the cosmetic formula to form an extremely potent carcinogen called nitrosodiethanolamine (NDEA). NDEA is readily absorbed through the skin and has been linked with stomach, oesophagus, liver and bladder cancers.

Formaldehyde

Formaldehyde is a colorless, strong-smelling gas that presents a health hazard if workers are exposed. You can be exposed to formaldehyde if you breathe it into your lungs, if it gets into your eyes, or if it is contained in a product that gets onto your skin. You can also be exposed accidentally if you touch your face, eat food, or drink after using a product containing formaldehyde without first washing your hands. It can irritate the eyes and nose, and cause coughing and wheezing. Formaldehyde is a "sensitizer," which means that it can cause allergic reactions of the skin, eyes, and lungs such as asthma-like breathing problems and skin rashes and itching. When formaldehyde is in a product that gets sprayed into the eyes, it can damage the eyes and cause blindness.

Federal OSHA (Occupational Safety & Health Administration) and State OSHA programs continue to investigate complaints from stylists and hair salon owners about exposure to formaldehyde while using hair smoothing products such as: Brazilian Blowout (Acai Professional Smoothing Solution, Professional Brazilian Blowout Solution), Brasil Cacau Cadiveu, Keratin Complex Smoothing Therapy (Natural Keratin Smoothing Treatment, Express Blow Out, Natural Keratin Smoothing Treatment Blonde)

Isopropyl alcohol

Isopropyl alcohol is typically found in hair rinses and finishing sprays. Isopropyl alcohol is used to give hair more shine, but over time, it can be very drying. (It's a petroleum based substance that is commonly used in wood lacquer and antifreeze.) It can cause headaches, dizziness, nausea, and abdominal pain. It is also used for massages and by athletic trainers to treat skin and muscle groups, hence the term rubbing. It has a drying effect on the skin and causes blood vessels to dilate; its distinctive odor is associated with doctor's offices, since it is used to clean the skin being prepared for an injection.

The Good...

So, we have identified a few of the bad ingredients in shampoos. What are the good ones? Listed below are just a few of the natural ingredients and terms that are most commonly found in shampoos, conditioners, lotions and creams. Most of these ingredients are products which are sold separately, and can be purchased in your local health shop or farmers market.

Aqua
Aqua is the Latin term for water. It is the scientific term used when listing ingredients for cosmetic. Water is normally listed as the primary ingredient in hair care products. Most products can contain between 50% - 90% water.

Shea Butter
Shea Butter is one of the creamiest, multipurpose moisturizers on the planet. This is a great for Used for moisturizing and softening the hair and skin. Shea butter varies from yellow to white in color. Shea butter can be found in West Africa It has many benefits from muscle fatigue to stretch mark prevention during pregnancy.

Glycerine
Glycerine also called glycerol is present in all lipids (fats) whether animal or vegetable. It can be derived from natural substances by hydrolysis of fats and by fermentation of sugars. There is also research indicating that the presence of glycerine stores up the skins natural protection by filling in the area known as the intercellular matrix and by attracting the right amount of water to maintain the skins moisture.

Aloe
It's no secret that Aloe Vera is good for your hair and scalp. Aloe Vera acts as a natural hair conditioner and can be used in place of chemical based conditioners. Using shampoo made with aloe

vera, or mixing one part of your own shampoo with two parts aloe, can help regulate oil production, according to AloeSajten.com

Vitamin E

Vitamin E has many other properties that maintain health and has long been used both internally and externally. Vitamin E has been shown to help with the growth of hair as well as preventing hair loss and has great moisturizing benefits.

Wheat Protein

It is very important for the hair to have protein, as well as moisture. Hydrolyzed Wheat Protein greatly increases the hair's ability to retain moistures, adds volume to hair, reduces the hair's porosity, and improves smoothness. Hydrolyzed Wheat Protein is able to repair the hair.

Silicone

Silicones have been a topic of controversy being labeled a bad ingredient, however this is misinformation. There are two types of silicones, water soluble and non-soluble silicones. Water soluble silicones can be washed away with water. However non-soluble silicones are exactly the opposite and require sulphates in order to be washed out. An ingredient with 'cone' as an extension contains silicone. Ingredients labeled: amodimethicone, or lauryl methicone copolyol, dimethiconol contains silicones. Silicones give products a slippery, glossy feel without being greasy. Silicone can be found in hair polishers, conditioners, and products that control frizz. It protects the hair from climatic conditions and moistures too.

Cosmetic Terms

Hypoallergenic
Hypoallergenic is used commonly in the cosmetic industry which simply means that it is less likely to cause an allergic reaction.

Organic
Organic refers to living things produced in a natural environment without the aid of man-made synthetics. Unfortunately, because the government has failed to step in and enforce the federal organic law, the marketplace has been flooded with synthetic chemical personal care products that are masquerading as organic. Ensure you look at the ingredients on the product as a precaution.

Fragrance Free
Fragrance free implies that the original scent has been masked as it may be deemed an offensive odor. People purchase fragrance-free products for a variety of reasons. In most cases, people buy them because they are sensitive to odors; pregnant women, people taking certain medications, and some individuals in a natural state are simply extremely sensitive to scents, with cosmetic fragrances causing discomfort.

Alcohol Free
Companies can label a product as alcohol-free if it doesn't contain ethyl alcohol (aka SD alcohol or alcohol denat), Methyl Alcohol or Isopropyl Alcohol, which all have negative effects on skin. But the same product can contain fatty alcohols, which can provide benefits to the skin.

Cruelty Free
Cruelty Free means that neither the final product nor its ingredients have ever been tested on animals. This is highly unlikely however,

as almost all ingredients in use today have been tested on animals somewhere, at some time, by someone - and could be tested again.

Be aware that labels that read "cruelty-free" and "not tested on animals" may not always mean what we think. As no government agency currently defines these terms, nor sets standards for their usage, it is left to each company to determine what its "cruelty-free" label means.

Fair Trade
Fair trade is sometimes substituted with alternative, responsible or ethical. Other organizations prefer the term 'community trade'. As most consumers understand it, this simply means paying producers-whether they be farmers manufactures or crafts people more money than they normally would receive for their goods and services, this is a key Fairtrade principle.

The goals of fair trade are: Improve livelihood, promote development, raise awareness, set an example campaign for change, and protect human rights.

Buying Fair Trade means you are helping farmers lift themselves out of poverty by investing in their farms and communities, protecting the environment, and developing the business skills necessary to compete in the global marketplace. Ingredients such as Shea Butter, coca, tea, coffee which are just as common in hair products are examples of fair trade. Buying Fair Trade Certified products, improves the livelihood of the poor and marginalized workers in the developing world.

www.fairtrade.net
www.lfat.org
www.bafts.org.uk

Chapter Two

Do You Lye?

Do you Lye? For sistas at some point in their life, there 'Lye's a dilemma .To stay natural or relax their hair. How much research do sistas undertake when considering whether to chemically process their hair, was keeping it natural also an option.

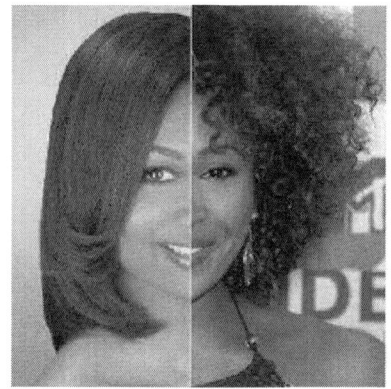

Sistas let me give you the 'heads up' on what those vulnerable strands are being subjected to when you choose to put a relaxer or texturizers in your hair.

What are the effects of chemical hair relaxers?

Relaxers, perm, straightening cream, creamy crack, the white stuff, are just a few of the names that are commonly used to describe this so called hair 'treatment'. The product does not in fact 'treat' your hair: it will eventually 'spoil' it!

Lye, also known as Sodium Hydroxide, or Caustic soda, the compound: NaOH (Na=sodium, O = oxygen, H = Hydrogen or OH = Hydroxide). Sodium Hydroxide is commonly used in drain cleaners and oven cleaners and is a potent chemical that is corrosive and damaging and very harmful when it comes into contact with human tissue. Ooooh, ouch!

Chemical burn via hair relaxing is self-inflicted and commonly unintentional cause of hair loss, scaring, and scalp damage. With the number of options for hair styling and treatments, hair loss due to chemical burns has become a common complaint.

In my research I came across an article published by the American Journal of Epidemiology Hair Relaxer Use and Risk of Uterine Leiomyomata in African-American Women January 10 2012.

"Studies show that there is a link between hair relaxers and uterine fibroids, as well as early puberty in young girls..."

"Scientists followed more than 23,580 pre-menopausal Black American women from 1997 to 2009 and found that the two- to three-times higher rate of fibroids among black women may be linked to chemical exposure through scalp lesions and burns resulting from relaxers."

Women who got their first menstrual period before the age of 10 were also more likely to have uterine fibroids, and early menstruation may result from hair products black women and children are using, according to a separate study published in the Annals of Epidemiology last summer.

Three hundred African American, African Caribbean, Hispanic, and White women in New York City were studied. The women's first menstrual period varied anywhere from age 8 to age 19, but African Americans, who were more likely to use relaxer, also reached earlier than other racial/ethnic groups.

While so far, there is only an association rather than a cause and effect relationship between relaxers, fibroid tumors, and puberty, many experts have been quick to point out that the hair care industry isn't regulated by the FDA, meaning that there's no definite way to fully know just how harmful standard Black hair care products really are.

Fibroids are tumors that grow in the uterus. They are benign, which means they are not cancerous, and are made up of muscle fibers. Fibroids can be as small as a pea and can grow as large as a melon. It is estimated that 20-50% of women have, or will have, fibroids at some time in their lives. They are rare in women under the age of 20, most common in women in their 30s and 40s, and tend to shrink after menopause.

According to US studies, fibroids occur up to nine times more often in black women than in white women, and tend to appear earlier. The reason for this is unclear. Also women who are overweight may be more likely to have fibroids. This is thought to be due to higher levels of estrogen in heavier women."

Love Your Natural Hair

In 1999 the American Journal of Epidemiology released a publication, Chemical Hair Treatments & Adverse Pregnancy Among Black Women In Central North Carolina

"Several studies suggest that toxic chemicals in hair products may be absorbed through the scalp in sufficient amounts to increase the risks of adverse health effects in women or their infants. Some of the affects are low birth rate and premature delivery. The studies were on black women and the affects their hair relaxers might have on their unborn babies. Sodium hydroxide, ammonium, and formaldehyde are just a few named chemical ingredients that can penetrate the scalp skin and enter the body of the mother and unborn baby".

These are serious adverse affects that should not be taken lightly, however some sistas who use chemical relaxers appear to be very blasé and as a result they are potentially risking their health.

Relaxing the hair breaks down the protein component in the hair. It breaks down the natural hair pattern so that the curls are straight.

Women who have opted for No lye, feel that it is a safer option, wrong! It is still a chemical based product with the intention of breaking down your natural bond in order to make it straight. The no Lye does have a slightly lower pH level and it has been reported that it is normally used on people who have sensitive scalp, as the burning sensation is not as intense. It may be easier on the scalp however; it is harder on the hair. Common complaints are brittle dry fragile limp hair; relaxers are the most drying chemical process that black women can do to their hair. The compounds in no lye relaxers are calcium hydroxide, guanidine hydroxide, lithium, or potassium.

For those women that are using 'Curly Perm', be warned, this is not the 'getting off lightly' option. The main active ingredient that is used in 'Curly Perm' is Ammonium Thioglycolate.
Toxnet, the 'Toxology Data Network' reports: the human toxicity report tested several women who were exposed to Ammonium

Thioglycolate, and also did studies testing for adverse affects of sodium hydroxide. The report revealed exposure to these chemicals can be harmful to the skin, irritate the lungs, and can cause 'allergic contact dermatitis.' In some cases inhalation of these chemicals has been known to cause asthmatic breathing, coughing, burns, blisters and blocked nasal passages in people who already suffer with asthma.

Just so you are aware of how damaging using chemicals on your hair are we will look at the pH. pH stands for Power of Hydrogen or Percentage of Hydrogen. The 7 indicates that its neutral. This scale assess how acidic or alkaline a product is. Dry hair has no pH. Only aqueous solutions have pH's. When hair is in an aqueous solution it normally has a pH that can fall between 4 & 6 on the pH scale. There are various strengths of relaxer; the pH also increases as the relaxer formula strength grows from sensitive scalp, to mild, to regular, to super strength. The higher the pH of the chemical relaxer, the greater the formula's ability to swell and lift the hair's cuticle. The more the shaft swells, the more damage to the cuticle. Relaxers made with Sodium hydroxide have a pH between 13.0-13.5!

pH Scale

0	7	14
ACID		ALKALINE

The Environmental working Group, published an article back in February 8, 2007, they did some research and found that 22 Percent of All Cosmetics May Be Contaminated With Cancer-Causing Impurity. Guess what the first product on their list is...?

- **97% - hair relaxers**
- 82% - hair dyes and bleaching
- 66% - hair removers
- 57% - baby soap
- 45% - sunless tanning products

- 43% - body firming lotion
- 36% - hormonal creams
- 36% - facial moisturizers
- 35% - anti-aging products
- 34% - body lotion
- 33% - around-eye creams

On their website, as listed above, they also have a list of other products, some of which have been banned in some countries. Lusters PCJ, Pretty n Silky no lye, for children and adults is banned in Canada and in some parts of Europe.

Many black women, both those who now have natural hair and those that still relax their hair, still complain that relaxers cause, limpness, dryness, and breakage. I wanted to find out which relaxer kit brands use marketing slogans which are misleading. I went to my local store and studied the – false - advertising. The statements were so misleading that I felt it worthwhile sharing them with you, below: I have added my comments, albeit a lighthearted, parody of their claims:

Brand-Misleading Statements
My statement

Olive Miracle-Anti breakage
"it will be a miracle if we still have any hair left"

Soft & Beautiful-Prevents Breakage & Dryness
"We were beautiful before we put this mess in our hair, there's nothing soft and beautiful about sodium hydroxide"

Soft & Beautiful Botanicals-The Natural Choice for healthy looking hair.
*"Oh really SBB the **natural** choice would be to put a chemical relaxer in my hair!! Who you fooling boo...hmmm hmm"*

Pink Luster-Smooth Touch
"oh no you didn't PL, you know you already have a rep, you need to go back to the drawing board with that!"

Laila Ali-Ultimate Treatment For Beautiful Hair
"The ultimate treatment would be natural ingredients, not a crispy scalp."

Olive Oil- Built in protection-
"I'm sure there is enough ammunition in this product to really do some damage to my innocent strands of hair! Oh Yes we will need protecting, agreed!"

Dark & Lovely- Strength,
'you got that right, I found the strength to come off the creamy crack,... now I'm free, thank the most high"

Motions-Intense Nourishment, "
"The word is not nourishment I think you mean malnourished."

Dr Miracles- Enjoy the Tingle
"Enjoy the tingle!! That is the understatement of the century, you mean enjoy the burn!!! Burn baby burn...tingle don't produce scabs honey."

As you can see from the above statements made, these brands and slogans are full of *creamy crack*!

Some of our Sistas will admit that they limit their choice of activities, because they are more concerned with the effect that perspiring, or dampness, will have on their hair, than to be free and enjoy themselves!

I will be the first to confess, that there were certain facilities that I would avoid, so as to keep my relaxed hair in check. Sometimes I would wait until the re-growth would appear before I participated in those extra-curricular activities. I was very dedicated to going to the gym though, and would ensure I got my high intensity work out every week. There are so many stories of how some women have allowed their hair to limit or dictate what social activities they will expose themselves to, for fear of moisture! I have learned to accept and embrace the transitions that my hair makes in certain environments. I don't let my hair be all consuming in terms of putting restrictions on my activities, or participating in events, for fear of my hair regressing to its natural state. This is a journey about growth and acceptance.

Hair Raising Experience

I attended a natural hair gathering hosted in Atlanta Georgia, I met some wonderful ladies who were happy to be interviewed and answer some questions and share their hair experiences.

Did having your hair natural or relaxed affect your relationships with partners, friends, or work?

Did having your hair relaxed or natural limit the types of activities you participate in?

Danielle had a relaxer from the age of 11 years old and then used a texturizer for 5 years. In 2005, she decided enough was enough and did the big chop and went natural. Her main style was a press out. She had been pressing her hair out so much so that she had to do another big chop, as her hair was breaking. So from February 2012, she did another big chop. She informed her husband that she was going to go natural but with an afro. Her husband questioned her- "do you mean an afro, afro?" Danielle explained she was going to be natural. Her husband said he was a bit apprehensive about her new hair style. However, a few months of being natural she said her husband absolutely loves it!

Dasha owner of Love Locks& Curls, has been natural for 6 years and has noticed that since she has been natural that she seems to have attracted more conscious, intelligent, men.

Tania, Youtuber and mother of two, has been natural for three years. When she did have a relaxer she didn't feel that it limited her in anyway. She still took part in activities and didn't have an issue with getting her hair wet. When she decided to go natural her husband would playfully mock her, waving the 'black power' fist on the odd occasion, but now she confesses he can't stop touching her hair. When she did decided to go natural she felt that her natural hair was limiting her success in her current job.

So one day, she thought she would test it out, and decided to do a 'press out' style for work. She wore her hair like that a few times, not long after, she was given a promotion. She then went back to her natural her style once she received the promotion. After some deep reflection about her working environment, She decided to leave the company. Shortly after leaving, she was hired by another company who accepted her just the way she is a natural beauty.

Felecia, 42 year old Business Analyst. In her spare time she likes to exercise, listen to music, surf the web, travel, try new restaurants and shopping! Felecia has been natural for one year. She had been relaxing from a teenager. She admitted that when she had a relaxer she tended to avoid working out until a few days later so that her hair wouldn't shrink. Her ex boyfriend preferred the natural hair styles however, Felecia at this point in her life would continue to relax her hair. After that relationship dissolved, she stop relaxing her hair, and now wears it natural. She is now in another relationship and met her current boyfriend who loves her natural hair, and is looking forward to seeing her grow.

Nylon 32 years, expressed that in the moments leading up to hot passion, that she would jump out of bed and head towards her side cabinet to reach for a...no...not that...........her headscarf.

"No I'm not about to waste my money and several hours in the beauty salon, for my man to put his hand all up in my hair, and

Love Your Natural Hair

he doesn't pay for it! No, He needs to keep his hand away from my head, & on my a**, (she laughs...) he knows the rules".

Kitoy Johnson glamour model, & Dancer, also known as 'The body' has been in several music videos including the rap duo sensation 'Outcast'. She shared a particular incident with me that led her to go natural. Kitoy was on tour with 'Outcast' for the song 'I like the way you move' video. She explained that being in the music industry it was common to get her hair styled by professional onsite hairstylist. Kitoy had relaxed hair and wore weaves that were bonded into her hair. The style that the stylist was trying to achieve was a teasing effect (back combing) for the video shoot. Three weeks later, she attempted to remove the bonded weave, which was tangled due to the teasing, which left her hair badly damaged with severe breakage, so she decided the only way to save her hair was to cut it all off. Her hair styles from that point on were pressing out the front of her hair and wearing half wigs until her hair grew back. With patience and perseverance and the support of her husband she has successfully achieved long thick, healthy natural hair.

Kitoy expresses "When I wore wigs, people thought it was my natural hair. Now I wear my natural hair, people think I'm wearing a wig!"

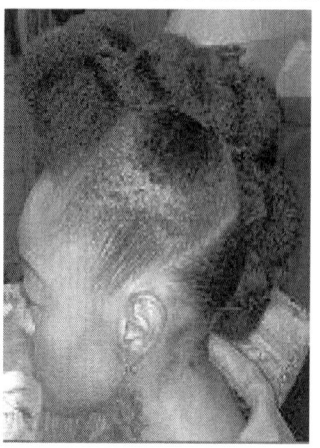

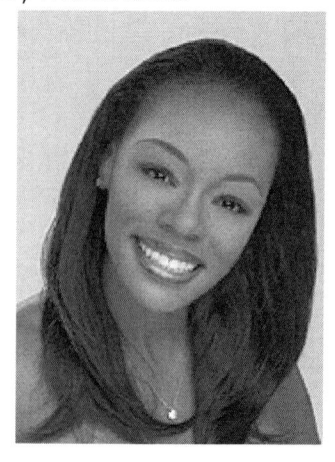

Youtuber: Kitoy Mowhawk

Kitoy's Philosophy: "I don't compete, I create"

Kissi Kurls

Cameron, age 12, and Angelina, age 11 years, are sisters, they attended the hair event with their mother Tania who wanted them to be in an environment with other natural sistas. They were happy to share with me what it is like to have natural hair whilst at school.

Initially when they first got their hair relaxed it was shoulder length, and gradually it kept breaking, getting shorter and shorter. Eventually, they were encouraged by their mother to go natural, and they agreed. Tania explained that the schools that the two girls go to the majority of the students are white, and her friends were curious about natural hair. They recall an incident while they were on the bus one day, one of the other children was teasing her about her hair, two pieces of her hair were upright and one of the children shouted out she looked like a devil. Occasionally they made sheep noises too. However, with the strength of her sister mother and aunt who were both natural, she remained self assured. She explained that the taunting soon stopped as the same girl seem to show an interest in her hair stating that she liked her hair. They told me that most of her friends had natural hair, however, they never wore their hair out they had it in braids most of the time. So one day she decided to bring a book into the school called 'Curly Girl' to help encourage the other girls. She was so surprised at the huge interest from her classmates, even her teacher who was also natural read the book. The girls told me that they enjoyed all the positive comments and responses they get from fellow classmates and the public by wearing natural hair.

Obsessions or fear based on our hair can potentially affect our relationships. Do not allow fear to run and ruin your lives. Below are the thoughts of some women who express their concerns about their hair and relationships.

~The following statements have been recorded from live interviews and have been paraphrased.

www.KissiKurls.com

Love Your Natural Hair

"On my Second date, the man I was dating told me he liked me, but didn't like my weave, and hoped that I would consider a natural style, so I kept my weave and got rid of him, he met me with the weave and already his trying to change me"

~ *Courtney B- Teacher*

"I wear a relaxer and have done for many years. Recently I have been feeling neglected by my friends who have decided to go natural. I feel like I am the odd one out as they are always talking about their progress with their natural hair. Socially things have changed too they are always going to hair events, doing track or going to the gym doing all these activities, that we never did before. I do not like sweating out my hair and they know this. I don't do too much exercise apart from walking. Am I being selfish?"

~ *Lisa Brydea Johms-Youth Leader*

"I recently shaved my hair (big Chop) BC. My mother has strongly advised that I put on a wig before go out with her in public. This has really upset me, it's like she is ashamed of me or something, and it's just hair, after all I am her daughter. I was feeling great when I cut my hair. Since she has made that statement I have felt self conscious, I love her but she is not the most tactful person. I wish she would get over it already."

~ *Tina Rogers, mother*

No Lye I'm Natural

There is also a social pressure for black women to conform to the western ideas of what their media considerers to be beautiful. We are constantly bombarded with images in the magazines & on television of long straight shinny fly-away hair blowing in the wind. These images have been in our magazines and televisions screens for decades. Is it no wonder, that when we reach our teenage years that a chemical relaxer is the first application that most girls want to try?

It is not uncommon to hear that some women may have been chemically processing their hair as early as childhood. What is disturbing to me is that in some cases, their parents choose this method of dealing with their child's hair. The child is not consulted or too young to understand the implications and may not be given a choice. Children are still growing; their hair follicles are still maturing and therefore still developing. Putting such raw, harsh chemicals on a tender child's head can lead to long term side effects that will eventually damage their hair, their scalp and more.

Is relaxing your hair for some black women, a form of an initiation from childhood to adulthood?

In hindsight, I think subconsciously it was for me. I was reluctant but curious to find out, if relaxing my hair was going to be the magic potion, was this the dream? Was my life going to change, because I relaxed my hair? Would my hair now blow in the wind and cover my eyes so I can't see? Will I be *head and shoulders* above the rest, just like the girls on the relaxer kit? Will my hair ever be the same again??

It was the mid 90s, weaves, relaxers and braids were very popular. I was a late starter for relaxing my hair compared to other girls in my age group, I was seventeen years old.

I was ready to be initiated: 'to cross the burning sands' (which is the initiation into a sorority). I was to withstand, for as long as I could, the burning sensation of the chemical relaxer on my head that made me feel like my scalp was on fire and brain was being cooked. I would have major dilemmas like: do I eat or do I do my hair?

I now had a 'date' with the salon. It would be every other weekend; this 'date' was intense. I would have to wait 5 hours before I was seen, and I was paying for and sharing my date with fifty other women! It seemed to me that someone else might be getting a benefit from this relationship but I was sure it wasn't me!

This sorority was more like a religion. I had to practice this ritual every week and put money away for the 'tithes'.

I was in the sorority, my hair fell flat and shiny on caressing my neck, although I now had length, my hair had lost its thickness; compared to my natural hair it felt limp. I was agitated by the scabs at the nape of my neck from the chemical relaxer; this was never mentioned on the warnings on the box or in the adverts. My hair looked like it had all the life sucked out of it. My Natural hair had volume and now I had to recreate that volume! However, I was now straight. Wasn't that the 'mane' thing?

Kissi Kurls

I was in the sorority, called the 'straight & sleek' I had made a pledge to maintain an image that, I was told, would potentially open more opportunities, increase my popularity, job prospects and possibly be adored by more men because I was straight. Now, all those things had happened, but not because I relaxed my hair, but because I showed perseverance, I took pride in my inner and outer beauty and continued to be a proactive and confident black woman.

I learned to conform, fit in and relax with everyone but I was bored, and tired, everyone looked the same. Although I had fun with the relaxer it came with a cost, one that was soon to be named frustration. It was time for a change. I had been bombarded with images of Europeans standards of beauty. African emperors and empresses are visions of beauty also, yet they are still not the forefront in the media. The Most High created us in his own image and likeness as perfect beings, to be loved and to show love, if we were all meant to look the same, then there wouldn't be variety in the world. The sorority I feel proud to be a part of now is 'No lye I'm natural'.

Ask yourself why do I choose to chemically relax my hair? If any of these statements listed below are similar to your responses then I would like to suggest that the responses given may be the result of conditioning, and low self esteem. If you have not taken the time out to love you, learn you and examine you, well, there's no greater time than the present. If you tried to go natural briefly and found yourself reaching for the 'creamy crack' it could be that you have not had the right guidance and technique on how to manage your beautiful hair.

I interviewed some women as to why they did not want to go natural. Here are their responses:

www.KissiKurls.com

"My sister's hair is better than mine and I don't want to embarrass myself with this nappy hair. I am the only one in my family that has this nappy hair, so I relax it, and if I have babies and they have this hair I will relax theirs too."

"I think them girls are brave, I will be too afraid that I will not be attractive, lord knows I need me some weave"

"I have been wearing a wig for 6 months I have alopecia, in hindsight I wish I had gone natural, maybe I could have saved some of my hair."

"I would only go natural if my hair was long, but it isn't so that's that!"

"I would like my wife to be natural, I keep advising her to get rid of that ridiculous weave, and do something with her natural hair, her hair is beautiful and so is she, but she said jokingly, I only want her to be natural so that she's not attractive to other men? I wish she could see what I see..."

I was really shocked and sad upon hearing some of the responses to going natural, I was stunned in fact. What follows are some of the most common responses that I have heard. Subconsciously, these women have developed a dislike for their hair and have adopted a mindset that something is inherently wrong with their natural hair, but this couldn't be further from the truth.

Negative/self-defeating thoughts	Positive/affirmative thoughts
I don't have good hair to keep it natural	A hair texture/type is neither good nor bad. Hair can only be healthy or damaged. The terms good and bad are terms imposed by those who wish to create a hierarchy between and within different racial groups. There is beauty in every racial type
If I go natural family and friends will think I'm not beautiful	When you learn to accept your natural beauty, others will see the beauty in you
I'm not skilful with my hair, it always looks messy when I do it	One step at a time, you can do it, put your mind to anything and you can achieve it
Natural hair will not suit me, it's only For pretty girls	The hair you were born with suits you, therefore you can be a natural beauty

In my profession as a counsellor, and a Natural Hair Transitional Adviser, the statements on the left column are statements that I have heard time and time again. I recognize such statements as non-supportive beliefs.

Integrative Therapy is the modality I prefer to use, which simply means the collective use of counselling models learned. One of the behavioral models that I would use for someone who presented these distinct concerns would be Rational emotive behavior therapy (REBT). Rational emotive behavior therapy is relative when we look at some of the misconceptions, thoughts, images, behaviors, beliefs and attitudes of some sistas regarding their natural hair. The basic assumption of REBT is that people contribute to their own psychological problems as well as to specific symptoms by the way they interpret events and situations. REBT uses an A,B,C model that examines behavior, attitudes and self statements.

Let's look at the previously mentioned statements:

"I don't have good hair to keep it natural"
This statement I would class as a negative automatic thought (NATS)

'I'm not skilful with my hair; it always looks messy when I do it'
To not even start a task because of a feeling of being incapable to complete them to the desired standard (perfectionism).

'Natural hair will not suit me, it's only for pretty girls'
Overgeneralizing: Labeling, and thus undermining the self

'If I go natural family and friends will think I'm not beautiful'
'Mind Reading', thinking we know what others think. Jumping to conclusions, predicting a negative outcome and then encouraging it to happen by telling oneself it will (auto-programming).'

The premise of this model is that the individual uses a set of principles and tools that will aid them through life by applying them whenever they need to find solutions to given attitudes, thoughts, beliefs and behaviors and resolve them through changing the mind set to a more realistic, positive and supportive belief system.

Mirror Mirror On The Wall

Client Case Study * Jasmine Krama

Background

Jasmine Krama is a client who was referred to me, for Natural Hair Transitional counselling after she had attended a natural hair exhibition and was considering going natural. She revealed to me that there were some issues about her hair that were holding her back from transitioning from relaxed hair to natural hair and wanted to address them. She informed me that she had already spent over $150 thinking that this would help her address the poor condition of her hair by purchasing many of the hair products on sale at the event. She had received some advice from the vendors and tips from other sistas who were natural but felt overwhelmed and expressed that she felt anxious but also excited. She described looking at all the different natural hair styles, colors and textures she had witnessed as a 'beautiful scene'.

Jasmine had become tired and fed up with the condition of her hair after years of relaxing and the relentless amount of time and money spent on trying to make it grow. She had dyed her hair almost every color of the rainbow and was amazed that she still had hair on her head.

Jasmine had been relaxing her hair since she was 13 years old and she was now 38 years of age. She remembers having thick, afro hair before she relaxed it. Her grandmother maintained her hair, by styling it in braids.

Love Your Natural Hair

She had been raised by her grandmother together with her brother whilst their mother pursued a career abroad as an international lecturer. Her grandmother taught Jasmine and her brother to learn to love, respect and accept themselves and be proud of who they were. Jasmine recounts the numerous conversations about wanting to look cool like the other girls and get her hair relaxed and have long straight hair, however, her grandmother advised her not to put chemicals in her hair. She remembers pleading with her grandmother but her grandmother stood firm and said that she would have to wait until she was old enough to work and pay for the relaxer as she was not paying for it and reminded her that she was beautiful the way she was.

Unfortunately, her grandmother died, whilst she was still quite young and Jasmine was devastated. She felt lost and as time passed, without the reminders from her grandmother, felt more and more unattractive. Her mother returned from working overseas to take care of her and her brother.

During this time her mother was their sole guardian and she tried to re-establish her relationship with the children, after so many years away. However Jasmine felt that she was now a stranger.

One day, she told Jasmine that she wanted to surprise her with a mother and daughter day trip out. Jasmine recalls feeling excited as she entered the hair salon. Her mother had, at that time, made a statement that Jasmine said played in her head several times a day. Her mother had said "I want to make you look beautiful; I brought you here to get your hair straightened.' Jasmine recalls this time painfully. She feels: 'my mother thinks I must not be beautiful!' This made her feel sad, however, she also recognized that she would finally be able to go to school and prove to her class mates that she was cool, straight and now as beautiful as they were.

Throughout her teens and then adult years, Jasmine admits that she spent an excessive amount of money and time going to the hair dressers trying different hair styles. She visits up to 3 times a week her favorite salon. She describes feeling frustrated, helpless, depressed, and suffered from low self-esteem and still feels unattractive. She just wants to look and feel beautiful. She admits that, having seen images of black women on advertising posters and in the media who have long, straight hair, she was trying to replicate their look. She has tried various hair styles so that she could replicate that very first feeling she had when she initially walked into a salon, in which she had her hair relaxed. She states, "I want to feel beautiful again".

Analysis

Having reviewed this case study we can apply the ABC model (see below) to see how Jasmine has come to behave the way that she does and to see how useful REBT can be as a way of gaining further insights.

Rational emotive behavioral Therapy uses the ABC model:
- A = Activating Event
- B = Belief/thought
- C = emotional and behavioral Consequence.

Acting Event - what are the events past and present that triggered Jasmine's thoughts or feelings at the time?
1. The advice from the vendors
2. Excessive visits to the salon
3. When her mother took Jasmine to the salon
4. Grandmother had died
5. Wanted to feel and look cool going to school

Belief - what were Jasmine's thoughts when the above acting events occurred?

1. Felt overwhelmed and excited about going natural.
2. The frequency of visits to the salon will make her feel and look beautiful
3. Felt her mother thought she was not beautiful
4. Grandmothers death led her to feel unattractive
5. Straight hair makes you look cool and beautiful

Consequence - How did Jasmine act or feel when she had those beliefs?

1. Spent lots of money on products
2. Jasmine felt frustrated and helpless when the condition of her hair did not improve
3. Having straight hair made her feel she would be beautiful
4. Felt lost
5. Considering going natural due to the damage and expense of having relaxed hair

She expressed that she felt sad, unattractive and was suffering from low self-esteem and depression and was trying hard to impress others. She had wanted to feel beautiful by frequent visits to the hair salon and trying to look like the models in the posters and in the media. She has become frustrated and is suffering emotionally and financially because of this.

Conclusion

There were many insights arising from our consultation that led Jasmine to look at the core of her issues. This has resulted in her being able to confront the issues that have plagued her for so long which led to her feeling insecure and ultimately holding her back from her inner desire to go natural.

The multiple events previously stated had a major impact on Jasmine emotionally and had been troubling her for years. She did not know how to communicate her feelings of hurt to her mother. There were also other concerns around the death of her Grandmother. Jasmine spoke of feeling that she had lost a part of herself when her grandmother died.

Changing her hair and trying to make herself 'beautiful' she was subconsciously trying to bring her grandmother back and also trying to please other people around her and to gain her mother's approval.

When we look at Jasmine's case we can ask ourselves whether the beliefs highlighted are justified by the Activating Event.

One of the approaches of REBT would be to reflect on whether the beliefs are justified or are based on erroneous assumptions or thinking errors. In the case of Jasmine we see an example of 'Mind Reading' making assumptions about what people are thinking. Her beliefs may be justified and accurate beliefs but they may also not be. It is important to clarify whether the situation and the evidence justifies the beliefs and then decide upon how to move forward once that has been done.

At the time of writing this book, Jasmine is 9 months into her natural hair transitioning phase and she is enjoying her transformation from relaxed hair to natural hair. She admits that it is one of the most significant and challenging journeys she has taken and tells me that she wants to eventually be an ambassador and inspiration for other black women.

"I look in the mirror I see me, I am beautiful, yes Grandma, I am beautiful!" Jasmine Krama

*for confidentiality reason the name used is a pseudonym

Hair sacrifice

You have to know why you are deciding to go natural, if its just a phrase then it won't be long before you relapse.

Whatever, the initial reasons for resorting to chemically processing your hair, the fact remains that the chemical used in chemical relaxers are so damaging that if you were to put a can of coca cola in Sodium Hydroxide it will disintegrate in less than four hours. Some women can sit for up to 30 minutes with this chemical on their head! A splash of relaxer in your eye can lead to blindness, also the inhaling of this chemical after long periods of time can damage your lungs and have an adverse affect on the body. Let's not forget the skin irritations' and the burns. Hair is essentially a dead protein; damaged hair lacks the active cells to repair itself. Unfortunately, lye hair relaxers strip the hair of moisture, and can burn or break the hair shaft. If the relaxer gets down to the scalp it can kill it at the root and can lead to bald spots. Now with all of that said, you would think that would be enough to conclude that it would not be an option for straightening the hair, however for many women it's a sacrifice their willing to take at all costs.

After years of chemical processing, some sistas can end up with no hair on their heads. There is nothing to manage at all! On top of that, the money that is spent on the relaxers is not even invested back into our own community. I watched the documentary named 'Good Hair' by Chris Rock, who interviewed a few, public figures, including the Reverend Al Sharpton about the Black hair care industry. The Reverend talks about black women: 'combing their exploitation, combing their oppression, attaching it, or hanging it up on the night stand'. He also states, 'If we can't control what nobody else's uses but us, that is real economic retardation' He makes the critical observation, however, his statement would carry more weight if he, himself, chose not to wear a relaxer, a product which is the target of his critique!

Chris Rock interviewed Mr. Dudley, who owns Dudley Cosmetology University and has a manufacturing plant worth over 100 million dollars, he is said to be one of only four black owned relaxing manufactures in this industry. It is estimated that black women spend in the region of half a trillion dollars on hair care! The sad thing is not a penny of it benefits our community.

There are people in the media who have had bad experiences with relaxers they are not exempt, if anything public figures, increase their risk of hair loss and damage due constant change of hair styles, which have to reflect the persona of the characters they play. Excessive hair styling puts pressure on the hair which will eventually have its consequences. Below are some women who have suffered or are currently suffering with hair loss.

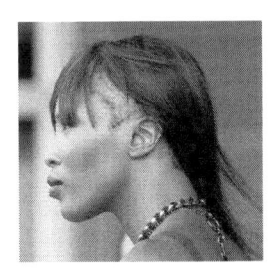

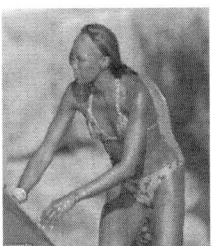

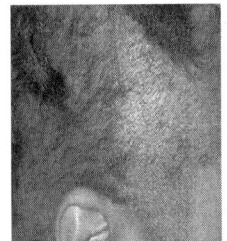

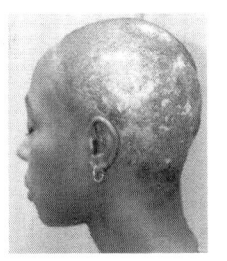

In these two pictures you can see Namoi Campbell with receding hair line. Oprah Winfrey has experienced hair loss. Oprah openly talks about the relaxer from hell that left her bald as a news anchor in Baltimore. She was lucky to have recovered!
Interview with Chris Rock: http://www.oprah.com/oprahshow/Chris-Rock-Feels-Oprahs-Hair
Oprah hair loss story: http://www.oprah.com/style/Oprahs-Hair-Nightmare-Video

Love Your Natural Hair

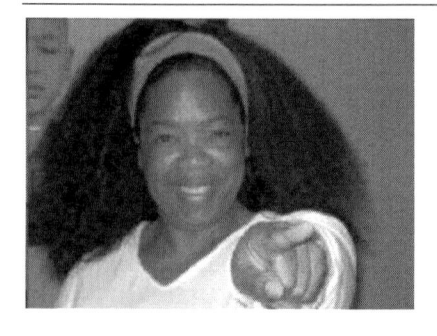

Oprah posts a picture of her Natural Hair pre-pressed or curled.

Oprah was tweeted, are you wearing a weave? Her response was "This is not a weave, this is my hair,"

Serena Williams

Champion extraordinaire, 'Serena Williams' changing hairstyles seem to be taking a toll on her hair. Recent photos show the 31-year old sporting a bald spot, a telling sign that she is likely suffering from a condition called traction alopecia.

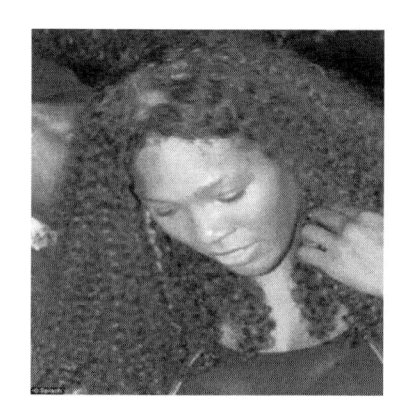

Salt & Pepper

Salt & Pepper very popular rappers back in the 90's, shared their hair story on Chris Rocks 'Good Hair'. First glance at the a symmetrical hair style which came about because a chemical relaxer that was put in Peppers hair fell out leaving one side of her hair bald. She confessed to coloring the bald spots with pencil and now can be seen sporting wigs and weaves.

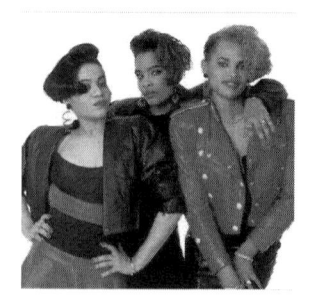

Hair Loss

They say hair is our crown and glory an important part of a women's identity. So many styles to choose from, long, short, kinky, curly, straight, braids, cornrow, twists, weaves, bantu knots, threading(banding) locks, wavy, highlights, low lights full color.

So what happens if you are one of those millions of people who suffer from alopecia?

Hair loss can be very traumatic especially for women that have been diagnosed with permanent hair loss. For some women, looking in the mirror is a constant reminder that they are suffering with a disease. Some people may think that there is no help for them if they lose their hair, whether it be temporary or permanent. It can be an emotional and testing time. It is important that you seek expert advice and consult a specialist.

As I write this book I can see that I am very lucky to have all my hair on my head and am in good health and I give thanks for this. With the regular or frequent weaving, braiding, relaxing, dying, gelling, crimping, tangling, and pressing, eventually those delicate strands of hair will finally break.

The worst case scenario is that you may even suffer with complete hair loss, in which case, your only other option will be to wear a wig, embrace the baldness, or, use a scarf. I can identify with hair loss, as I noticed that some years ago whilst I was natural I was having a few small bald patches on my head. I had to reflect that this might have been the result, if not of my genes, then of my actions a few years earlier and the use of hair chemicals.

At the time I didn't consult a dermatologist although I really should have. I just assumed I was going to get through the 'bad patch', so I just ignored it. In an effort to have control over the few patches, I decided to cut my hair to about four inches and start again. My hair has grown back since and is in a better condition, although cutting my hair wasn't necessarily the cure.

If you see visible signs of hair loss do consult a doctor, especially if you are losing large amounts very suddenly. Hair loss can happen to anyone, for several reasons including, but not limited to illness, cancer medications, work, emotional stress, childbirth, thyroid disease, and more.

Alopecia

I came across some information about Alopecia and the various types, conditions, causes and ways in which to encourage growth. This condition can happen at any age. It is stated on the Alopecia American Autoimmune website that there are 2 million people who have some form of alopecia. The most common type of alopecia are:

Alopecia Areata
Hair loss Bald patches occurring anywhere on the body.

Alopecia Mucinosa
A type of alopecia which results in scaly patches.

Alopecia Totalis
Total loss of the hair on the scalp.

Androgenetic Alopecia (AGA)
Also known as male pattern baldness; It is a thinning of the hair to an almost transparent state, in both men and women. It is thought to be a hereditary form of hair loss.

Alopecia Universalis (AU)
Total loss of all hair on the body.

Traction Alopecia
Traction alopecia is usually due to excessive pulling or tension on hair shafts as a result of certain hair styles. It is seen more often in women, particularly those of East Indian and Afro-Caribbean origin. Hair loss depends on the way the hair is being pulled. Prolonged traction alopecia can stop new hair follicles developing and lead to permanent hair loss.

Anagen Effluvium
This hair loss is generally caused by chemicals such as those used to treat cancer. Initially, it causes patchy hair loss, which often then becomes total hair loss. The good news is that when you stop using these chemicals the hair normally grows back (usually about 6 months later). Other drugs also can cause hair loss. Many medicines used to treat even common diseases can cause hair loss.

Scarring Alopecia
A form of alopecia, which leaves scarring on the area of hair loss.

Telogen Effluvium
A form of hair loss, where more than normal amounts of hair fall out. There is a general 'thinning' of the hair. Unlike some other hair and scalp conditions, it is temporary and the hair growth usually recovers.

'Mane' cause of hair loss

The most common type of hair loss experienced by Black women are:
- Improper use of products that chemically alter the natural hair texture
- Applying new relaxers over previously relaxed hair
- Excessive hot-pressing, curling or blow-drying
- Gluing hair in during the weave process
- Chemical or heat burns to the scalp
- Combining permanent color with other chemical hair treatments
- Braiding hair to tight -Pulling of hair
- Stress, post traumatic stress

Styling Bald Hair

What will you do when you lose your hair?

If you suffer with hair loss and are looking for ways in which to remain stylish, there are many hair pieces, wigs, hair adornments to choose from. Wigs come in all styles and colors. A wig made of real hair could cost between £800 and £3,000, or more, and it requires more care than you give your own hair. Most women choose synthetic wigs. They look and feel good, need very little attention and care, and cost much less £30 to £500. You can also wear a head scarf, if you want to change your style there are so many colors, patterns, textures, and styles to choose from, and they look fabulous! There are some great hats too, baseball hats or summer hats. I would recommend if you are bald maybe place a stocking cap or cut up some old tights to place on your head before you put on a silk or stain scarf, otherwise the scarf may slide off. Alternatively, you can buy a Pashmina or cotton scarf, natural fibers will not irritate your scalp. You can also buy scalp pencils which help to fill in any bald patches. Start with light stokes to create the illusion of hair strands in the direction of the hair.

Remember, in cold weather you will lose a lot of heat through your head, so keep your head covered. In the summer ensure that you do not expose your hair to, too much sunlight wear a hat or cap. For fair skinned women, you may need to protect your hair with sun cream.

The other option is, you can just rock your beautiful bald head.

Encouraging Growth

If your hair loss is temporary and you see new growth, allow the new hair to come through without putting any stress on the hair, such as pulling from braids or cornrow. Allow for the hair to get to a significant length, before deciding to braid or cornrow the hair. Consult your trichologist for more specific directions and a growth plan for your new hair.

It is good practice to massage the hair occasionally, when accompanied by an essential oil this can be very stimulating and encourage growth, here are a list of just a few essential oils that encourage growth as well as other benefits:

- Lavender oil
- Rosemary oil
- Lemon oil
- Sage oil
- Thyme oil
- Lang Lang oil
- Cedar wood oil

Although it's upsetting to lose your hair, a diagnosis will help to begin the healing process which is the first step to helping you move forward. My role as a Natural Hair Transitional Adviser & counsellor is to help you emotionally & psychologically with your hair loss. I am able to empathize and guide you along your journey.

Love Your Natural Hair

I have personally found that having my hair natural feels rewarding, I'm constantly learning growing, being creative, resourceful, economical, and networking with like minds. Here are the personal benefits that I have experienced:

- Natural hair is a Point of discussion
- Recognition and compliments
- Have a lot more money to spend
- Stand out
- Natural Hair Networking events
- Looking at other aspects of your life that would benefit from being natural such as food, cleaning products, health
- Making my own hair recipes
- Inspiring, empowering and building with other women
- Learning, about my hair care and organic products
- Contributing & strengthening the economy

Having your hair natural means you can do so many styles, styles that you may not have even tried before. I recognize that this may be a big step for the newbie naturals, I was there myself several years ago however and I haven't looked back.

"Afro hair is not a problem, when one learns to accept ones natural beauty & stop looking for solutions for a problem that doesn't exist."

"Navigate your mind and your feet will follow"

"Great achievers have one thing in common; they take a small step before reaching their goal."

This Is The Hair

"Know that this is the hair you were born with,

This is the hair that your parents gave you,

This is the hair that you need to work with,

This is the hair that will protect you from climatic conditions,

This is the hair that will aide your beauty,

This is the hair your partner will stroke,

This is the hair that you have tried to suppress, straighten, and stretch,

This is the hair that has seen many decades,

This is the hair that has always came back,

This is the hair that will go grey one day,

This is the hair that will need to you to occasionally say...I love my natural hair."

Hairstory In Pictures

Our Young tender tresses, "*au naturalle*", siblings and I rocking our natural hair? Can u spot me? I'm sporting my 'Little House On The prairie' dress in dark blue.

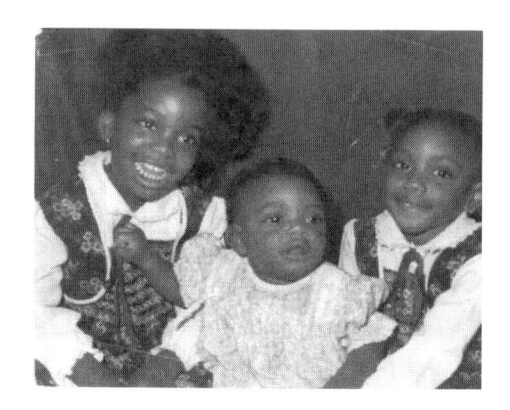

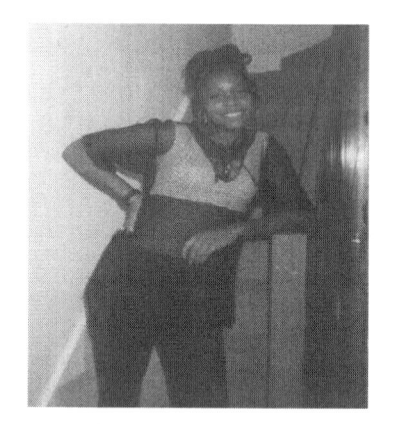

Relaxed hair my signature 90's hair styles.

Thick lengthy Relaxed hair, then my hair began to break.

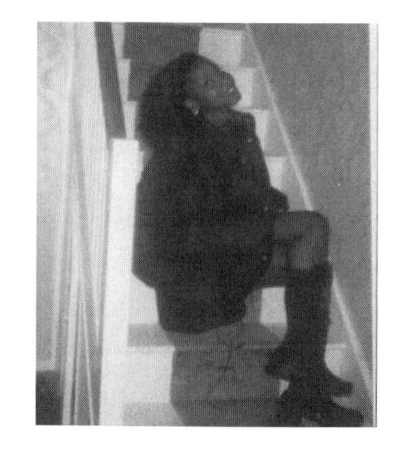

Kissi Kurls

Curly & straight weaves- not realizing my natural hair was the same body and length as the weaves!

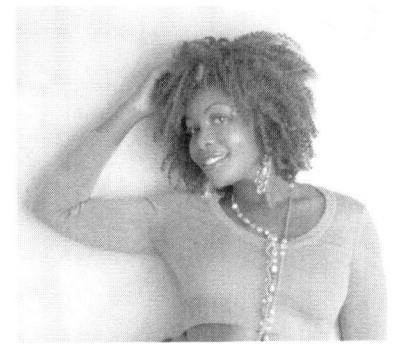

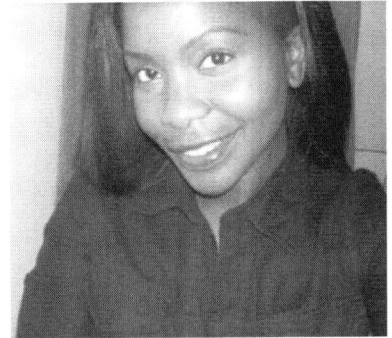

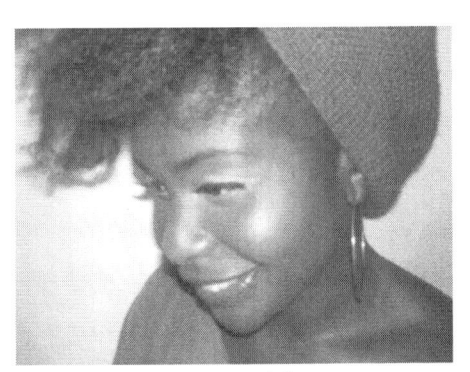

Accessorizing

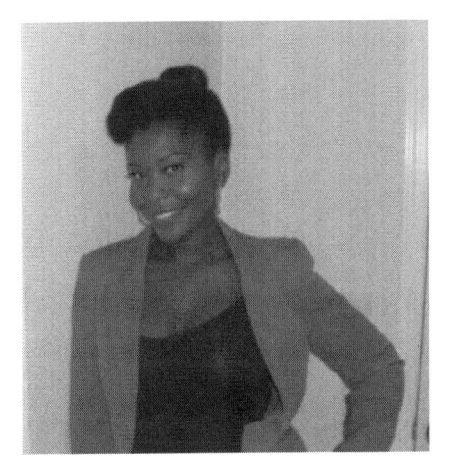

Who said natural hair can't be sophisticated!

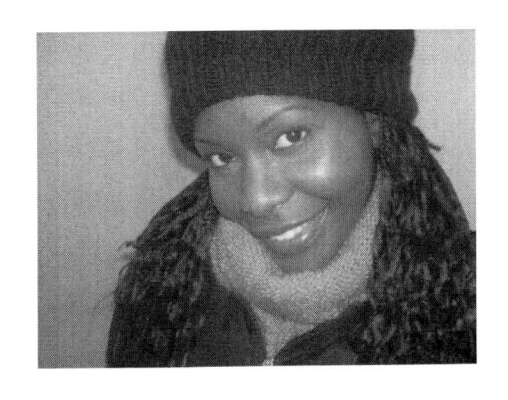

Extensions- winter warmer protective style

www.KissiKurls.com 117

Love Your Natural Hair

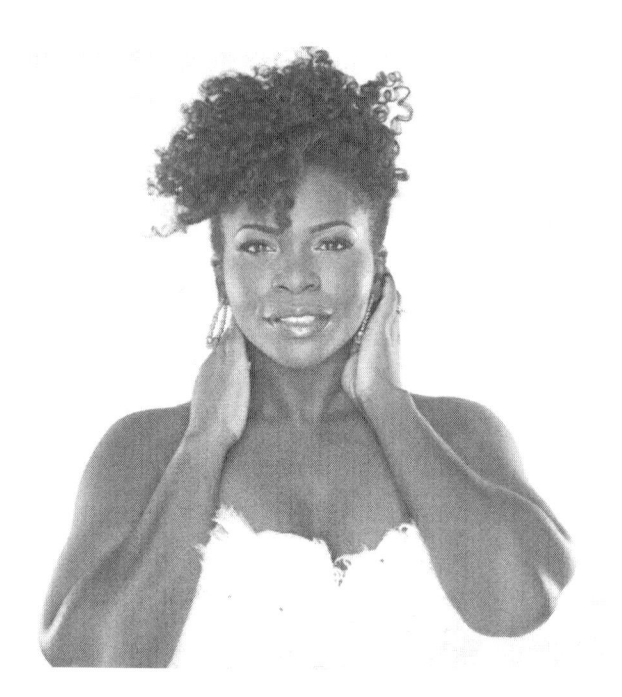

Natural hair up do

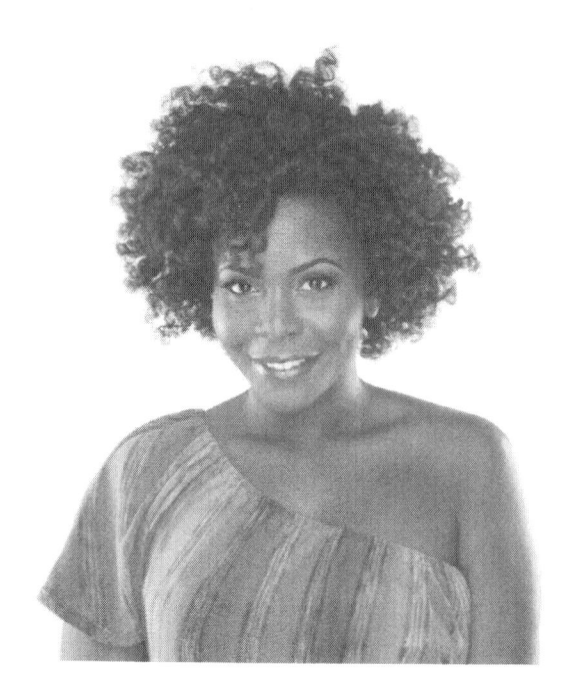

Loving my
Natural Hair!

www.KissiKurls.com

Chapter Three

Kinky, Curly, Coily, Tales

The following are stories from people I have interviewed and stories that I have come across that exemplify the beauty of having natural hair. I hope you will enjoy them, just as I did, when I first heard them.

Michelle Obama 1st Lady
"There's a picture in the oval office that we don't take down. The picture is of an African American boy who visited us along with his class on a school trip. The boy asked Barack, "Is your hair like mine?" Barack answered "yes".
Barack then bent down so the boy could feel the texture of his hair. After feeling the texture of Barack's hair he said, "Yes, it is like mine" and smiled. This is such a powerful image on so many levels; it's significant to us because this represents change."

Source: Steve Harvey Show

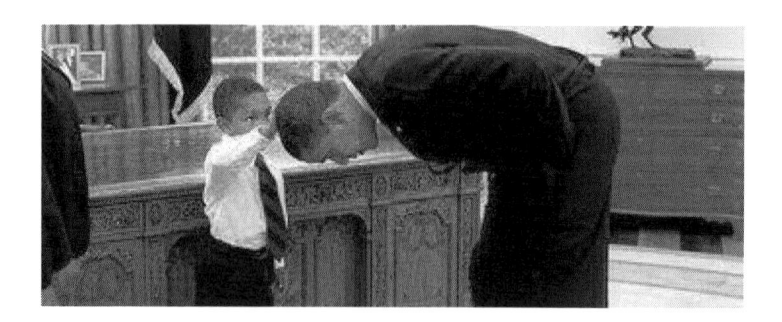

Amel - New York Entrepreneur & charity Raiser
"In 2002 I went natural. I had twists, people thought that I was a lesbian and some even tried to sell me drugs! Besides that My experience has continued to be positive. I wear my hair short I love wearing it short."

Laytoya Brown Sugar - *Natural Hair Stylist*

"When I wear my hair straight I get a different response from men. I get 'cat calls', whistles, and the approach is degrading and there is no respect. However, when I wear my hair natural, I get called queen, empresses, beautiful. It's more respectful and of high honor. Men are more attracted to women with their natural hair verses extensions or weaves, especially when you in a relationship."

"You can't change any situation if the root is not addressed no matter how you change it on the outside you will continue to produce the same seed."

Brenda - *Accountant*

"I'm originally from Tanzania; I wore my hair short all the time when I lived there. When we moved to the United States, I noticed that my hair was breaking a lot. I'm not sure if it was the water. So I started wearing wigs and weaves, and I think I liked to wear them because it made me feel like an adult, I thought this was more appropriate. Now I'm thinking about going natural, I think I'm going to give it a try, but I fear that my hair is a bit too thin, but I will try it and see."

Rhonda Lee - *Meteorologist*

When I read this article I was appalled at the way in which Rhonda Lee was treated. In my opinion Rhonda Lee's response to the Facebook comment was dignified, polite and articulate. However, she was fired from her job for responding to a Facebook comment made by Emmitt Vascocu he wrote:

"The black lady that does the news is a very nice lady. The only thing is she needs to wear a wig or grow some more hair. I'm not sure if she is a cancer patient. But still it's not something myself that I think looks good on T.V What about letting someone a male have waist long hair do the news what about that."

Rhonda Lee Responded:

"Hello Emmitt I am the 'black lady, to which you are referring. My name is Rhonda Lee; Nice to meet you. I am sorry you don't like my ethnic hair, and no I don't have cancer. I am a non-smoking 5'3, 121lbs, 25+ mile-a-week running, 37.5 year old woman and I'm in perfectly healthy physical condition. I am very proud of my African American ancestry which includes my hair. For your edification: traditionally our hair doesn't grow downward. It grows upward. Many black women use strong straightening agents in order to achieve a more European grade of hair and that is their choice. However in my case I don't find it necessary. I'm very proud of who I am and the standard of beauty I display. As women we come in all shapes, sizes, nationalities, and levels of beauty. Showing little girls that being comfortable in the skin and HAIR God gave me is my contribution to society. Little girls (and boys for that matter) growing up in this world need to see that what you look like isn't a reason to not achieve their goals. Conforming to one standard isn't what being American Is all about and I hope you can embrace that.

Thank you for your comment, have a great weekend, and thank you for watching."

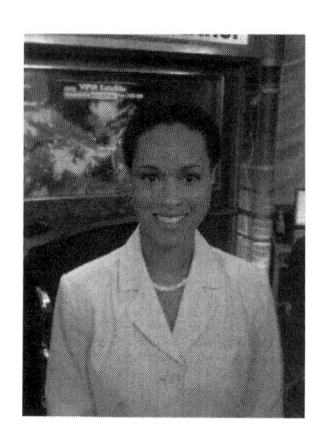

Rhonda Lee
Meteorologist
Source: www.huffingtonpos.com

Namoi Kissiedu Green - *Model, Actress*

"I'm 33 years old, and still having hair dramas!! It started when I was 16 years old. I decided to finally perm my hair myself!! I couldn't afford to spend money at the hairdressers and I knew most people did it at home. Both my sisters had really lovely long hair, and my friends at school all permed their hair and had that straight long look.

My hair didn't' really take to the perm maybe it wasn't the right strength as I had thick coarse hair. Anyway, this was the start of me perming my hair every month instead of every 6 weeks, and not just perming the roots, but the whole of my hair. I didn't follow the instructions and didn't really manage my hair properly over the years so it started to break. Over the next few years I started putting my hair in braids, weave and other styles but didn't have my natural hair out!! I became addicted to this long versatile look, the fake hair got me to the point where I would never give my hair a break. Once I would pull it out of a style, I would put it straight back in braids!! I would hate guys to see me with my natural hair, as I thought I didn't look the same (attractive) Like so many other women It became an addiction that I spent a lot of time and money on.

When I was in my early 20's, I finally had my natural hair for a few weeks (only because I couldn't find someone in time to do my hair before I had to go to work) The reaction I got was so good, everyone loved it, I was shocked and felt so good. I couldn't maintain my hair for long and started with the hair braids. I arrived in Australia and after a while I decided that I just didn't care what people thought. I think it was because there was less pressure to have your hair styled in a certain way, maybe because there were less black people here to really care. So, I finally went natural after a few years living in Australia I got married, and later fell pregnant. My friend permed my hair, when we finished I saw how long my hair had gotten, due to the hormones in my body- it's the best time for your hair, so I looked after it for a while then it started to break because I didn't, yet again maintain it. I didn't spend money at the hairdresser and kept perming it, so back in braids it went! A year on and my hair is totally broken!! It's got bad split ends and my sides had broken-off, so I decided enough is enough and cut it off short. A month of growing it natural it still needs to be trimmed and I'm still finding it hard to think of different styles but I know if I persist I will get the natural afro beautiful hair length that I want. My friends are also at this stage, so we are doing everything we can to grow it naturally, investing time and making our own hair products and researching how to grow our hair.

While modeling in Australia they didn't understand how to style afro hair so I put my hair in weaves a western style, to make it easier for them, but still there was so much drama because I could not pull up my weave or style it in a certain way, so I changed to a lace wig. On the day of the shoot, my lace wig lifted up and we couldn't glue it down, it was so embarrassing!! Years of doing the same thing, I'm now over it. I have decided if the modeling industry want to use me then my hair will be natural and they will just have to figure it out with my help.

I only hope that this time round being pregnant, I will stay true to myself and carry on this journey. There's so many inspiring women wearing natural hair, so I know I'm not alone, I have found out I'm having a baby girl, so how can I tell her to be proud of her hair, if I can't do the same, so this is my promise to myself."

Going Natural and proud. X

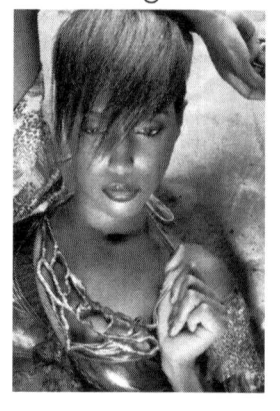

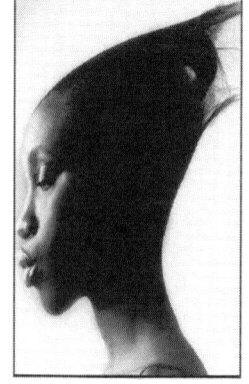

Maudelene - *Vegan catering company*

"I was sitting on the train with my best friend. We both had our children next to us. My daughters hair is long curly and natural, people assume that she's bi-racial but she's not. They make this assumption because she has long curly hair. My friend's daughter's hair is also natural and was braided at the time. The people on the train were directing compliments to my daughter at how beautiful she was and how lovely her hair was. They completely ignored the other child who was also beautiful, but because she didn't have long curly hair they ignored her, this really upset me. So I purposely kept smiling at my friend's daughter and reassuring her that she too was beautiful."

Deborah Sagira

"Since being natural for 2 half years, my 15 yr old son always comments how he like my hair and does not like me with a weave. Cornrows are nice, extensions, braids are okay, as are twists, but my natural he loves."

Jamilah

"I have been natural since 2004; my family and friends were like why did you lock your hair? I responded, its hair I can choose to do something different cant I. A lot of my people don't understand that you want to embrace the essence of who you are."

Al-Yasha - *Philosophy Professor at Spelman College*

"In 1989 I locked my hair, I was a swimmer on the water polo team; it was easy for me to deal with. I remember my grandmother, saying that she liked my locks now that they were long. However when I used to visit my grandmothers cousin, she would say she wanted me to use a pressing comb for the sides. I thought this was funny!"

Love Your Natural Hair

<u>Shanarae</u> - St Croix Virgin Island - *Dancer, Choreographer, Activist*
"In 1997 I went natural to attend Clark Atlanta University; I wanted a more natural lifestyle. I initially transitioned with braids it is very liberating I was ecstatic. When I went back to St Croix to visit my family after going natural, my family was shocked. My dad said 'you need to comb your hair; I liked it when you had a perm. For the most part I have had positive responses to my natural hair people say your hair is so thick, and I wish I could go natural. I got my mother to go natural, at first she questioned it, but the fact that she is natural I feel like I have accomplished something and I feel I did good in the world."

<u>Ayanna</u> - *Elementary Teacher*
"I have been natural for 22 years, I went to a barber to get my hair cut, I asked the barber what she thought, she said " if you want to look like a boy!" It seems to me that the response is more positive if you have long natural hair than short. I collected my things and left the barber and went to the barber a few doors down. When I walked in to the other barber I decided not to ask his opinion, I realized I was seeking validation from other people. I decided to feel secure within myself."

<u>Yvette</u> – *Self-employed, and Jazz Enthusiast*
"I went from relaxed to natural, relaxed, then back to natural and I'm going to stay natural, I have been natural for two years. I want a Healthier lifestyle and want to do something else with my time after spending so many hours in the beauty salon. After two years of being natural my mother still says every now and again" is that how you're going to wear your hair? "My experience has been so positive; I get positive comments all the time."

Pat - *Legal Analyst*

"I am natural and free from the chemicals, it was the chemicals that ruined my hair, my hair used to be fairly long. I relaxed my hair because I was encouraged too; the relaxer kept breaking my hair. I went back to being natural and have been natural for 8 years. My husband without fail would take me and my daughters to the beauty salon every week to get our hair relaxed. I feel that he liked straight hair. One of my daughter's her hair is really long, and when she had it straighten he would glorify her hair, he did comment on my other daughter but because her hair was long and flowing he paid her more attention. My other daughter has gone natural, however my daughter with the long hair, wants to go natural but doesn't commit to it; however her daughter, my granddaughter loves my natural hair and as a result has gone natural too. I am no longer with my then husband who is ironically moved on to be with a lady with locks! My daughter with the long hair, I feel holds onto her straight hair, as I feel it is a form of an attachment to her father, who compliments her straight long flowing hair. My daughter is now married, and it appears that she may have attracted a man like her daddy, who likes straight hair. The irony is, that she is now ready to go natural, but her husband likes her hair straight and doesn't want her to go natural."

Liz - *Midwife, Doula- Dekalb Medical*

I have a few black friends, when I think of black women and their hair I noticed that the black girls with straight hair seemed to hang out with white people and the girls with more afro hair tend to hang out with a diverse group of people that's just what I have seen. My friend had extensions for a long time and seemed to be resettling with whether to go natural, which I didn't quite understand. She recently decided to wear her own hair and seems to be encouraging everyone around her to do the same. I think afro hair is so interesting, black women can do so many things with their hair, my hair is just straight and boring. When I think about this subject and why black women feel the need to have straight hair, I do feel a little sadness within me, because I feel.... did society do this to you, to make you feel that you were not beautiful, and that this was the only way to get ahead?

Esther Kissiedu - *Social and Digital Manager*
My natural hair story: "It's been just over a year since I decided to stop relaxing my hair. After 12 years of relaxing my hair I felt my scalp craved a break from the constant burning sensation that brought short time joy in the form of my silky locks. The first few months of not chemically straightening my hair felt good. I felt free. I hid my hair under weave and then twists and then back to weave and so on. Last week I took my hair out of extensions to let it breathe and I uncovered a tangled thick mess. It was painful as I tried to comb through the weeks of un-brushed hair, and even more painful when the hairdresser attempted the same thing. It hit me right then and there. When had I decided to go natural? I had made the conscious decision that I didn't want chemicals on my head but what I hadn't realized was with that came a defining moment, I would be entering a new hair care world. I'd be discussing what my hair type number was searching you tube videos on how to maintain natural locks. It's something I hadn't prepared myself for. I become aware of the divide that exists between the natural and relaxed. It feels much more then a hair choice but a life choice, one I'm not sure I'm ready to make. Yet suddenly here I am a year later in the transitioning stage wondering whether to continue with what I started or return to the ease of a relaxer. As my fro bounces freely and thickly I feel like I have made my decision..."

Dileane - *Human Resources, & singer*

Well, firstly I would like to say that there is one thing that really upsets me when I think about my hair. It was a negative experience I had with my hair. When I think of the times that I have postponed, cancelled, arrived late or was tired and frustrated, my hair was usually the culprit. In 2006, I was dating a guy I'd just met. He was a conscious Brotha. At that time I was wearing extensions and weaves. We had many a conversation, as you do, during the dating stages. I had butterflies in my stomach, so excited was I to have met him: intelligent, proactive and damn, he looked good!

We had a discussion about hair, he was encouraging me to wear a natural hair style, and I was up for it, and had arranged for an appointment to get my hair done before I saw him next. One day he asked me to come with him to look for a tuxedo for a work event. I turned him down! Guess why? My hair wasn't done! My appointment wasn't until the following week and I felt I couldn't see him with my natural, but 'not yet done' hair, so I cancelled on him. The following week to my shock and horror he died. (Raised voice)Why! Why! Why! Why! Why! We have to stop doing this, to stop making excuses and missing out on opportunities, love and happiness. We need to learn to accept who we are! I am so angry with myself. It's still painful... I wish I could turn back the clock, I really, really wish I could. I would leave my house bald just to have seen him again. Now he is no longer here.(Tearful).

I would not want anyone to do this to himself or herself. Don't let anything hold you back. I'm not going to make that mistake again.
I wear natural hair now and am grateful for his encouragement. If my hair is not done for work, an event, whatever, I just go anyway. I lost this amazing man and although it was seven years ago, I still shake my head in disbelief. I've cried and cried. Why did I meet him only for him to be taken away so soon? So, please do not make my mistake, live your life to the full. Don't let your hair get in the way of you achieving or being. Please, please! That's the message I would like to share with your readers."

Natural Hair Gallery

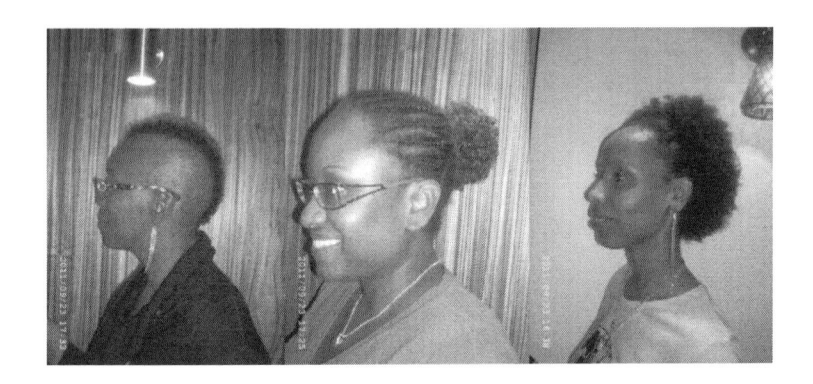

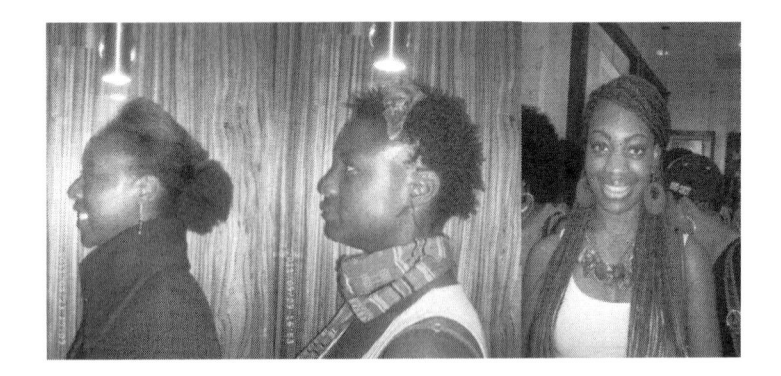

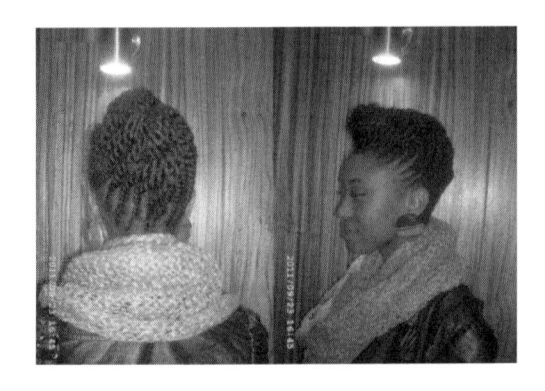

Kissi Kurls

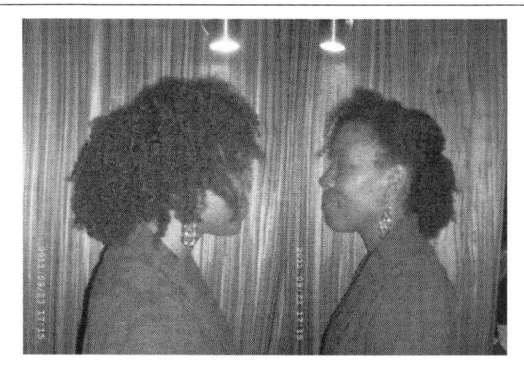

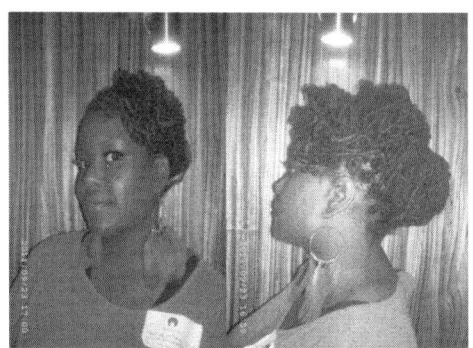

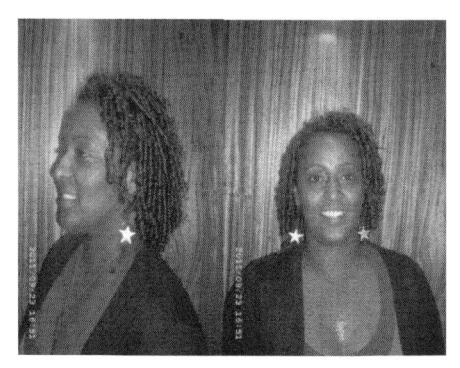

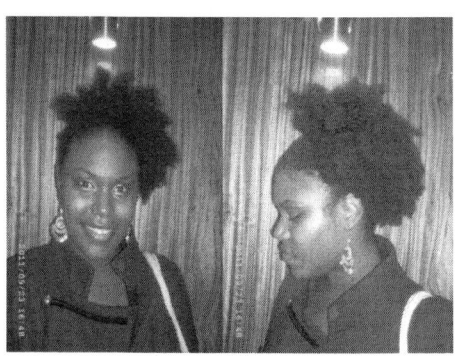

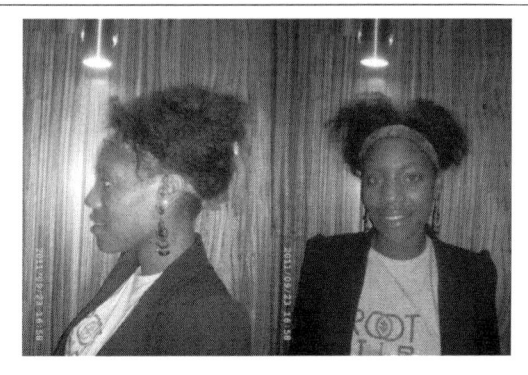

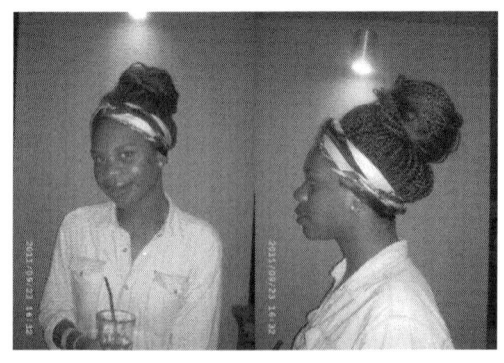

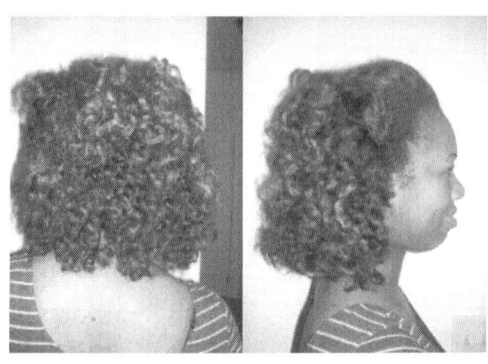

Love Your Natural Hair

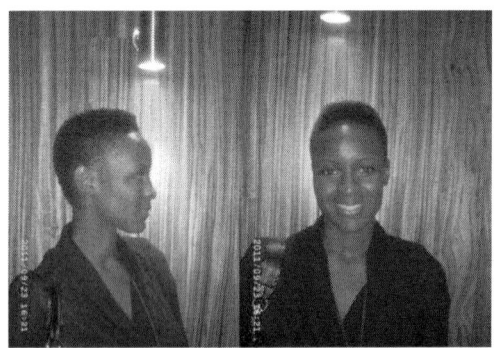

Kissi Kurls

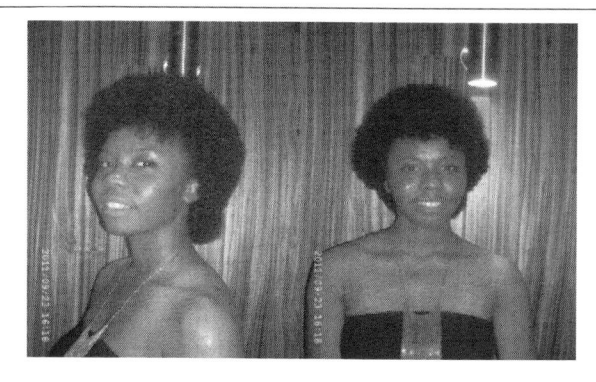

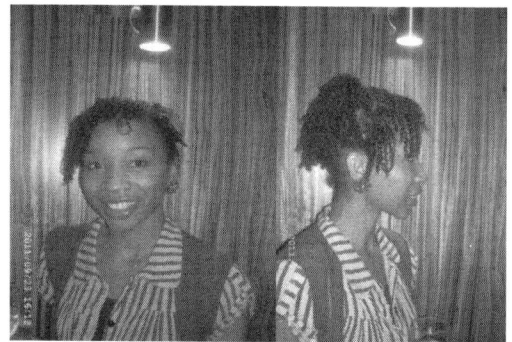

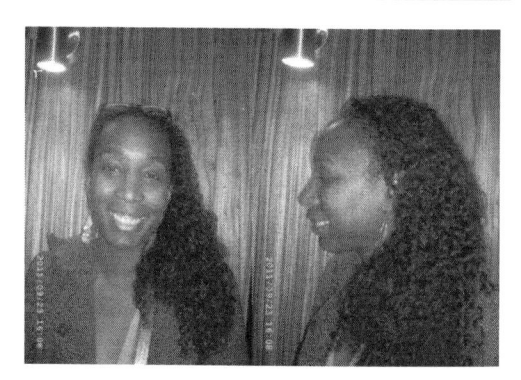

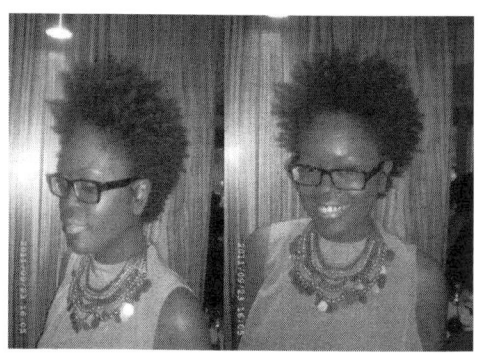

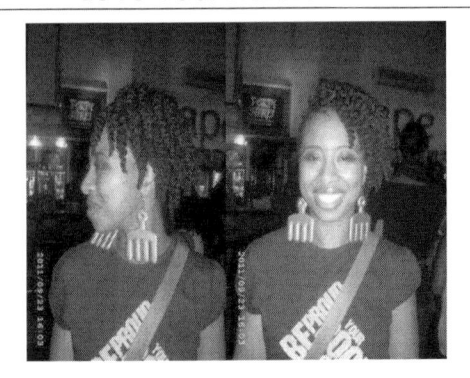

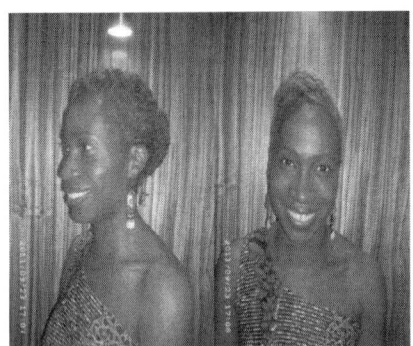

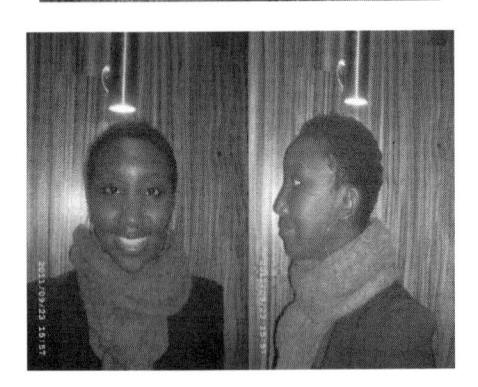

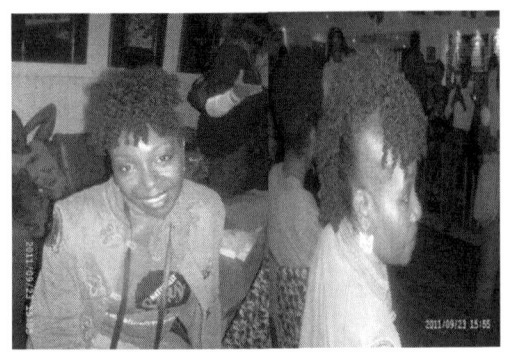

Love Your Natural Hair

134 www.KissiKurls.com

Natural Hair Questionnaire

I wanted to find out what members of the community's thoughts were on natural hair. So I went to my local shopping centre and interviewed ten 'relevant' people at random. These are the results below:

1. **Question:** How many men have seen their girlfriends/wife natural hair?
   Answer: 6 out of 10

2. **Question:** What is the most popular natural hair style?
   Answer: Puff, Twists, **Twistout**, Afro

3. **Question:** What is the common length of time to go without washing your hair?
   Answer: Once a week, **Every Two Weeks**, monthly

4. **Question:** How many girls with relaxed hair would consider going natural?
   Answer: Eight out of ten

5. **Question:** Do you like natural hair?
   Answer: Yes 9, No 1

6. **Question:** What were the most compliments/comments on average received in a month about natural hair?
   Answer: 20

7. **Question:** How many women have been inspired to go natural because of a friend/family member/colleague went natural?
   Answer: 7

8. **Question:** Do you use the Andre walker system?
   Answer: Yes 2, No 5, No Knowledge of it 3

The N.E.S.S. Hair Type System

I created The N.E.S.S Hair Type System based on the number nine. The number nine is the highest number in numerology. Nine is a very significant number. For example the gestation period of a baby is nine months, the Fibonacci spiral; a mathematical pattern found in nature, is also in the shape of a nine: sea shells are shaped like a nine. ; Nine-Ether expresses the combination of all existing gases and 9 is the highest number in mathematics. If you take a 9 volt battery and rub it against steel wool, it will start a fire; the minimum voltage for this ignition process is 9. There is a saying that a cat has nine lives; the nine times table answers all add up to nine. When you multiply any number by 9, then add the resulting digits and reduce them to a single digit, it always becomes a 9. For example: 6 x 9 = 54, 5+4 = 9; or 23 x 9 = 207, 2 + 0 + 7 = 9, and so forth. Afro hair coils in the shape of a nine. There is nothing coincidental about this.

So, with the aforementioned in mind, what is the physical reverse of 9? It's 6. The opposite of coiled hair is straight. So, descending from 9 is 8, 7, 6; six being straight hair. Again, the diagrams are purposely drawn in a circle. For a circle in degrees is represented by 360o: 3+6+0=9, and the semi circle is also 180 o 1+8+0=9.

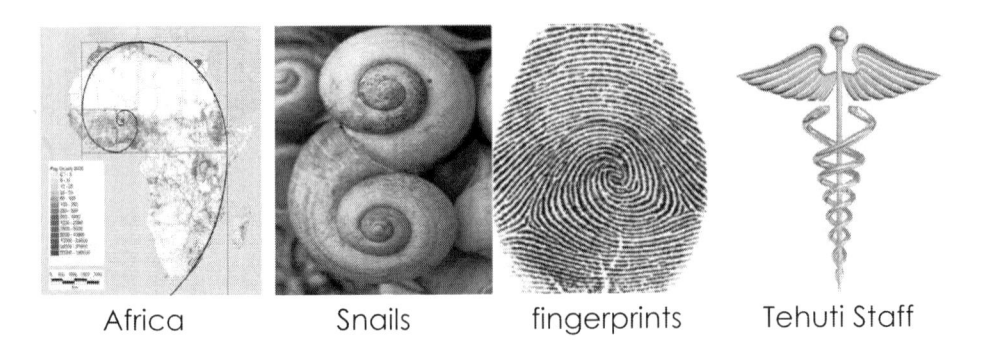

| Africa | Snails | fingerprints | Tehuti Staff |

The words, SPIN, SPIRAL, and SPIRITUAL share something in common: The supreme power spins, spirals, it is spiritual. The universe moves in spirals. The entire universe dances in spirals and rotations; everything in it reflects the 'SPIRaling, SPIRitual' essence out of which it is made. Your blood spirals through your veins, Plants spiral up from the soil, and kinky hair spirals out from the roots! Ball your hand into a fist and slowly extend each finger...

The 'SPIRal,' especially the 'Golden Spiral', is simultaneously the most profound motion and design in the universe and it is built into all life forms. The galaxy and the universe both rotate in a similar curved pattern. This was known to the ancient sages who worked with these curved patterns in nature which were thus held to be divine: as above, so below: an ancient knowledge.

The Caduceus is the staff carried by Hermes in Greek mythology. Hermes is equivalent to Tehuti in ancient Egyptian mythology. Tehuti is an Egyptian deity renowned for mathematics, medicine, writing, 'thought' and magic. The Caduceus or the staff of Tehuti is a symbol that is commonly seen as a symbol for medicine. The two serpents can be seen spiraling around the staff.

N.E.S.S Hair Type System Explained

N.E.S.S is an acronym for Nine, Eight, Seven, Six. The numbers in each section represent the hair type and texture which are: Coiled, Curly, Wavy and Straight.

Here is the first diagram below, 1 of 3. Going from nine to six the hair is straightening and the reverse, from six to nine the hair is curling.

Love Your Natural Hair

9 - COILED, OVERLAPPING CURLS
8 - CURLY, LOOSE CURLS
7 - WAVY
6 - STRAIGHT

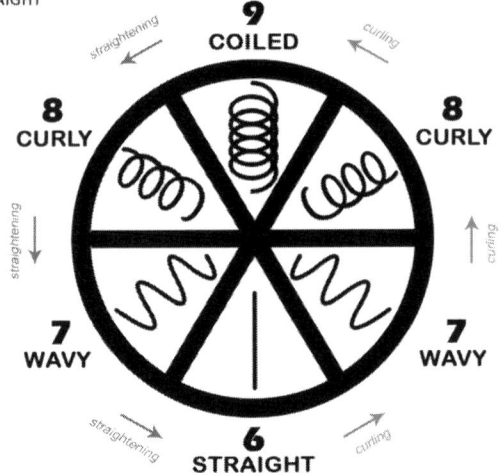

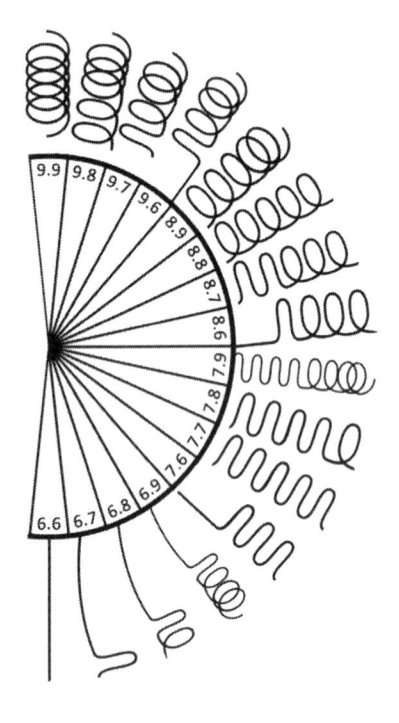

There are four categories within each section. Here is an explanation of how **The N.E.S.S Hair Type System** works. The hair type 9.6 for example is the least tightly coiled hair in the nine section. Some part of the hair maybe very loose almost straight, but not as straight as 6.6 which is in the six category and is bone straight.

I feel it's best to identify your hair type whilst its wet. If the majority of your hair is Coiled then your hair type will be in the Coiled category, if the majority of the hair is curly then your hair type will be in the curly category, if the majority of the hair is wavy then your hair type will be in the wavy category and lastly if the majority of the hair is straight then your hair type will be in the straight category.

138   www.KissiKurls.com

Kissi Kurls

Coiled 9	Curly 8	Wavy 7	Straight 6
9.9 All coiled	8.9 curly & coiled	7.9 Wavy, curly, coiled	6.9 straight, wavy, curly, coiled
9.8 coiled & curly	8.8 All curls	7.8 wavy, curly,	6.8 Straight, wavy, curly
9.7 coiled, curly, wavy	8.7 curly, wavy	7.7 All waves	6.7 straight, wavy
9.6 coiled, curly, wavy, straight	8.6 Curly, wavy, straight	7.6 Wavy, straight	6.6 All straight

This is **The N.E.S.S Hair Type System** in its entirety, from point 9.9 coiled hair to 6.6 straight hair.

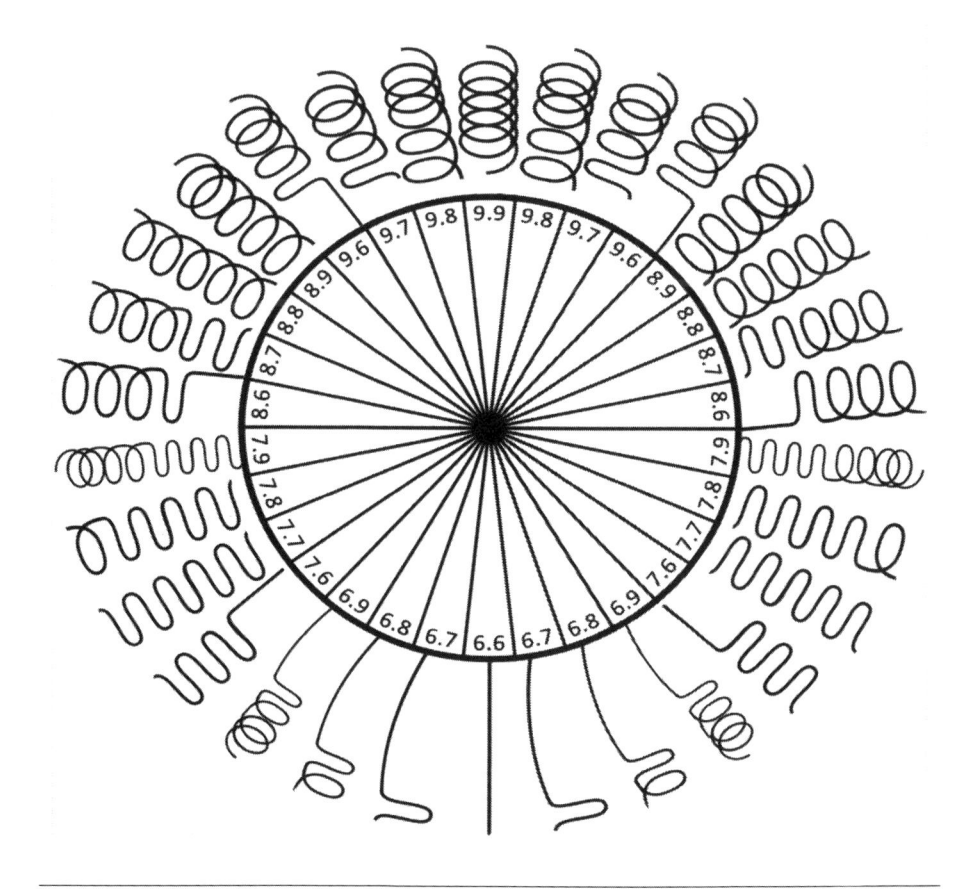

www.KissiKurls.com

Hair Type- Hype?

Within the Black community there is a fascination with hair texture. There are many hair types, as there are various shades of brown skin.

When making the decision to go natural there are a few questions that may come to mind. One of those questions maybe, what does my natural hair texture look like? What is my hair type? Some Sistas may be thinking, how do you not know this? Remember, that it may have been several years ago that some transitioners may have seen their natural hair, and in some cases they may have never seen their hair texture or know what hair type they are until they go natural.

I created **The N.E.S.S Hair Type System** to extend the range of hair types referred to, as I didn't feel that the current systems I encountered were a true reflection of the diversity of afro hair. When interviewing other naturals, they too were not so comfortable with the current hair types system. Some didn't understand the current systems and others didn't feel hair type coding was necessary.

I wanted to create a system that was simple, useful and purposeful. The beauty of **The N.E.S.S Hair Type System** is that it takes into account multi-textured hair. Afro hair varies from tightly coiled to lose waves. An individual can also have multi-textured hair on different areas of their head. I decided that I would devise a system that would incorporate the various textures which would also account for multi-textured hair.

Andre Walker's system has been criticized by some 'naturals' for being limiting. It does not take into consideration multi-textured hair and is limited to three categories in each section. Below is an article from Elle magazine, who have interviewed Mr. Walker and this is his response below in dealing with afro hair:

"Oprah's Hair Stylist pisses off Kinky haired folks
Andre Walker Oprah's affable stylist upset Sistas with natural hair by saying, "I always recommend embracing your natural texture. Kinky hair (however) can have limited styling options; that's the only hair type that I suggest altering with professional relaxing." ~Jan 7th 2013- Elle Magazine

Upon reading this statement, I felt very uncomfortable. I certainly was not going to use a system designed by someone who felt this way about afro hair. I felt inspired to create my own hair type system; one that would take into consideration the great variety of hair textures, together with a more diverse range of hair types. I feel that black women will appreciate that this system is designed with them in mind and has been created with love and appreciation of afro hair.

Our parent's genes have been passed down onto us. Therefore, it should come as no surprise that we inherit some of their fabulous genes, skin color, eye color, nose, and hair types. Two people coming together with differences will naturally conceive a child that inherits these differences and more. For example, my husband has four different hair textures on his head 9.8,7,6. I don't think he could quite believe it, until one day we went to the barber and the barber said he has never had to use 4 different shears on one head before. One of the shears the barber used was normally used for 6.6 hair type (straight hair). When we got home, I filmed his hair so that he could see the different hair textures on his head. This helped him to understand why hair, in certain parts of his head, was responding differently to pomades and shampoos that were applied.

Is Hair type, all hype? Here are some examples which show why knowing your hair type can be of benefit. There are some people who keep a track of their calorie intake. If you are trying to manage your weight or trying to lose weight this method will help you monitor your progress so that you can achieve your desired goal Weight. The same can be said with credit scores. How many of you know your credit score? Once again, it depends upon what you're trying to achieve. If you are trying to finance a property or increase your spending power then keeping track of your score will aid you in your quest. It's the same with hair type. It is beneficial to be aware of your hair type so that you know what the best hair products are for you. This way you can achieve the optimum results for your hair and have realistic style outcomes for your hair type. If you have 6.6 (straight) hair type and you put Jamaican castor oil in your hair this would saturate your hair as this oil is too heavy for this type of hair. As a result it will weigh the hair down leaving it greasy and potentially clog your pores which can attract dirt leaving you prone to a bad hair condition.

As for styling, someone with 6.6 (straight) hair attempting a twist out, will have a different style outcome when compared to a person with a 9.9 (coily) hair type. The 6.6 hair will need products with extra hold, such as extra hold moose, or holding spray, or extra hold gel as this hair type doesn't hold curls for very long. Whereas the coily, curly wavy hair type, is likely to need little or no holding product as these hair types retain curls.

Porosity

In conjunction with using The Ness hair type system, it's helpful to know the hairs porosity, Knowing how porous the hair is will help you to correct the balance of moisture using the necessary products and methods that will give you the best results for your hair.

A pore's ability to store liquid is called porosity. Porosity is dependent upon your hairs ability to absorb moisture past the cuticle layer of your hair, into the cortex layer.

Moisture loss occurs because the hair is more ready and willing to let the natural Moisture escape from the inner fiber into the atmosphere. Healthy hair is well able to maintain its moisture levels. Both porosity and moisture loss are a result of cuticle damage. Simply put, the cuticle layer is no longer tightly aligned and is no longer providing adequate coverage to the inner hair shaft.

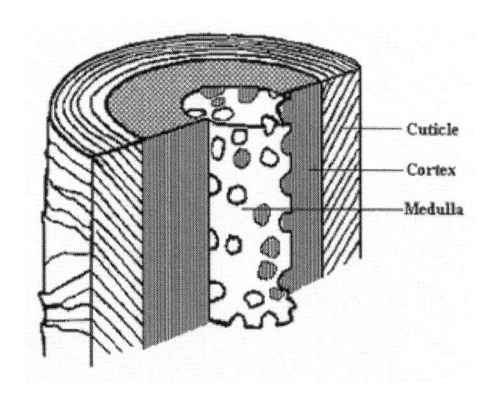

Hair becomes brittle when it has lost a significant degree of moisture. Cuticle cortex damage and the porosity that results from such damage, are the fundamental reasons that hair loses it softness and becomes straw-like in feel and appearance.

Love Your Natural Hair

Testing the Porosity

One way to test the porosity of the hair firstly, ensure the hair is clean and free from products then place the strands in a tall glass of water. Wait 5 minutes.

The results:
- High porosity – Your hair immediately sinks; your hair cuticle is open so it absorbs moisture easily.
- Low porosity – Your hair sits on top of the water; your hair cuticle is compact so it does not absorb moisture easily.
- Balanced porosity – Your hair sinks to the bottom of the glass slowly; your hairs porosity is balanced.

High Porosity

High porous hair, are raised cuticles that absorb moisture. The moisture escapes very easily, because the cuticle layers are open, therefore making the hair dry, brittle and prone to breakage. Hair styles such as twist outs, for example, tend not to hold, resulting in shrinkage.

Care

Highly porous hair requires the use of silicones, heavy oils, or butters to seal the moisture into the hair to avoid evaporation. Keep a spray bottle to hand to keep the hair hydrated. Apply a protein treatment, the protein from the conditioner will act to help fill in those holes and cracks in your hair shaft adding strength to help prevent breakage. Always finish off with a cold rinse to close the cuticles.

Balanced Porosity

Balanced porosity hair cuticles lay flat and absorb the right amount of moisture, it is neither resistant nor overly porous. Chemical applications are performed routinely and received well. Beware however, if considering a chemical process, this will change balanced porous hair to high.

Care

Try adding lite oil such as coconut or jojoba to your conditioner. Regularly steam your hair with your favorite conditioner and ensure you finish off with a cold rinse to close the cuticles.

Low Porosity

Low porosity hair cuticles layers are compact and lay flat, it can take a long time to dry, with some naturals waking up to damp hair the next day. When applying products the product tends to sit on top of the hair, leaving unattractive residue.

Care

Those with hair of low porosity should avoid thick creams or butters, as they will not be absorbed and leave hair feeling greasy. Try using a light, liquid-based product that will not just sit on top of your hair making it oily or greasy. Use a steamer or heat cap when deep conditioning your hair to lift the cuticle, so that the moisture can be absorbed Try using the *Cotton dry method. Use a cotton t-shirt, instead of a towel. See if it makes a difference to your drying time. Dry your hair as you would with a towel. Apply products to your hair when it is damp rather than wet, and finish off with a cold rinse to close the cuticles.

*Note: 'Hair plopping' is a technique using a cotton t-shirt. Apply necessary products for styling and then, using a cotton t-shirt ideally with long sleeves, wrap hair into a turban. When hair is wrapped up it will compress the curls for curl definition, (If you have short hair it will make it look shorter). You can leave the turban for as short as ten minutes to as long as overnight. Once removed you can air dry or use a diffuser on low heat. Ensure that you apply a protective serum throughout the hair. This is used also to prevent frizz.

Hair Doctor

Questions and answers with Hair Doctor Lisa Akbari

1.   What should people expect when they visit a trichologist?

"Well, the first thing you should expect is a full microscopic and physical examination. The microscopic examination should be done under several levels of magnification to check for density, scalp disorders and to check if your (hair) follicle is allowing for a true texture to emerge. Also you should get a recommendation of different practitioners, a dermatologist depending on the findings of the Trichologist. You also should expect the Trichologist to perform the microscopic and physical examination with a monitor in front, so that you can see what they are doing and so they can explain their finding and why you're having a particular problem.

You should expect a diagnosis which will tell you what's wrong and even a prognosis which will give you an idea of how well you will be able to improve. The Trichologist should give you a percentage as it relates to balding the percentages are based upon the ratio of follicles that are damaged or destroyed to the ones that are just perhaps blocked or ingrown. It is how much you can expect the hair to re-grow which is crucial. We also have coverage numbers, which tells you how much hair growth to expect. It is based on the percentages of strands that are all present that will offer coverage to the hair follicle that have been destroyed through damage or a hair follicle that has lost its ability to produce a new strand.

Each follicular unit is a pore and there are several follicles within each unit. Each follicle has one hair, so with the microscopic view, your trichologist should be able to tell you whether or not the follicle is functioning, or if the follicle has a blockage, so ideally you want that microscopic view."

2.   How important is it to visit a trichologist?

"It is crucial. I always tell my patients to do a home examination first and then do an examination with your stylist. At that point if you see that there are problems then consulting a trichologist is best. A trichologist can tell you what direction you should go in, whether you need to see another practitioner with a different background or whether they can help you with your particular problem.

If your Trichologist can treat your problem then it will be through a natural/drugless method or treatment. If the practitioner is a dermatologist-trichologist then he can write a prescription. Trichologist normally cannot write perceptions as they are not medical doctors but they can treat disease of the hair and its connection to the scalp. This will solely be dependent on their practice and their area of research."

3.   How regular should one schedule an appointment to see a trichologist?

<u>Stabilization</u>
"What I do with my patients when they come to see me is that I start out with what I call stabilization, the first part to my four part program. As Stabilization will be the first part, initially you may see the trichologist often maybe once a week over twelve weeks then after that you will go on to what's called maintenance."

<u>Maintenance</u>
"After stabilization your problem is pretty much settled. You should have stopped losing hair, your scalp problems are stable and then

you are ready to go into maintenance re-growth where you will actually grow the hair. You can begin to re-introduce chemicals, if you use chemicals, or begin to transition into natural if you are thinking about transitioning, or you can wear color. During this part or phase you will actually begin to obtain length to your hair. In cases where you have blockages then the trichologist may recommend specialized more advance treatments. During maintenance you will visit your trichologist every 4 to 16 weeks."

Prevention

"The next step or phase is prevention at this point your problems should be solved, you should have been able to maintain the stability that you achieved during stabilization, and now you want to prevent the problems from returning. Prevention is a bit like maintenance because prevention at this point is enabling you to maintain the hair you desire. You'll want to have a program that's going to determine how well you are going to manage your hair all year round. Many of you may need to see the Trichologist for hydrating treatments during the year, within some of the seasons. Keep in mind our scalp is skin and it will change during the winter spring summer and fall months. I like my patients to visit every season to see how the scalp responds to that particular season. A patient may only see the trichologist for a microscopic view/follow-up analysis, but may need treatments."

Extension Prevention

"Following prevention there is extended prevention which is what you do for life. My patients will be able to say "I know that I'm well if I have been able to stabilize my problems and now I'm no longer losing hair or having scalp problems; I have maintained stability and I'm preventing the problems from returning. What do I do now? "At this point I recommend that patients schedule an appointment once a year, for a physical and microscopic examination of their hair strands and scalp. This is a similar commitment to having a physical examination for your body once a year. In those cases where the scalp problem is chronic, then I would ask that the patient visits twice a year for a physical and microscopic examination. During that examination I will choose one of the seasons that are most challenging, in other words which season the patient notices a flare-up of scalp and hair dehydration, breakage, or itch. At that point I would provide a hydrating treatment that was appropriate for that particular season."

4. What advice would you give to someone who is thinking about going natural?

"The advice I would give is to consider your choices. You have to remember, when you are going natural, that God did not make a mistake in you having natural hair, that's the hair God gave you. Let it be something that you want, not something you are running from. Always tell my patients, that in some cases women who are transitioning are like women who are leaving an abusive situation. In such a situation they would run out of their houses, with bare feet, into the middle of the street and say, 'I'm free and now what do I do?' They have left the relaxer and now what do they do?

I have lots of patients that are 'natural' yet they don't know how to take care of their hair, so I would say to them that if they like straight hair then you should wear straight hair. And Remember, the pressing combs and strengtheners can cause damage but with the proper hair and scalp program care you can wear your hair straight using either technique. As an alternative, you may choose to texturizer your hair, which is a chemical treatment that removes some of the curl pattern and then one can use a roller set.

Just remember If you want to go natural I think it's a great idea but you really need to do the research and research a program on transitioning. Unless of course, you just desire to do the 'big chop' but because it's pretty traumatic to do the 'big chop' I would say it is better to transition. It is important to be sure it is something you really want to do and then make sure you also have a good re-growth management program.

Finally, look for a good natural hair stylist to help you , not one that just styles your hair but one who knows how to work well with people who are transitioning and who can take care of your hair and scalp during your transition, offering, advice on hair products and home maintenance That's crucial."

5. In your opinion what is the number one damaging product that black women should avoid?

"You want to avoid products that are not water soluble, in other words you want to make sure that whatever you use on your hair and your scalp has the ability to rinse clean from the hair and scalp, and not leave a residue. I call them clean products; clean products do not necessarily have perfect ingredients but these products don't harm the environment and they rinse clean from the hair. When you have a moisturizing shampoo or conditioning shampoo that's problematic, it means it causes cosmetic pollutants to develop on your scalp and hair, resulting in all types of problems which relate to your scalp and your hair.

Avoid the waxy products that will not protect the hair."Products that are waxy are not clean products, so often you find people using these products but eventually they will cause cosmetic build up. Avoid waxy products: products that don't rinse clean from the hair and scalp after the shampoo, such as heavy, greasy products. Oils are wonderful and should be used to seal moisture in your hair and scalp. Proteins will keep your hair strong but the levels must be balanced. There is a delicate protein and moisture level within the hair strand that must stay balanced. So I would recommend that you use a conditioner that has protein and moisture in its formula."

6. What are the benefits of having natural hair vs. relaxed hair?

"Your natural hair is you! It's a part of you, you are not your hair but it's a part of who you are. God made your hair, God makes no mistake. So just from that standpoint it's great to have your natural hair, you feel so good as a black woman with natural kinky hair or a woman of color because you have taken ownership of something you were born with. Now that's my opinion, I think it's a choice; I think God does not care if you have natural hair or relaxed hair. What's important to me is If I'm doing something that's wrong or harmful. I had a patient that said to me once, "I have relaxed hair, God told me not to relax my hair"
I said "hmmm" I thought for a minute and I thought well, if God said not to relax your hair, well maybe your right, she looked and she paused a minute and this is a patient who has been having problems with the relaxer and had damaged hair.

I said listen God does not want you to do anything that is damaging or is going to harm you so if relaxer is harmful for you, and you can't maintain or manage it or take care of your hair while wearing a relaxer then I believe for you, that you should not wear relaxed hair. Hair is dead once it emerges from our follicle, its dead cells keratinized, so it is very important for you to protect and preserve the dead fiber so that you can have body with your fro. If you want to wear your relaxer wear it, if you want to wear your hair natural wear it, but take care of your hair."

Chapter Four

Unique

Afro hair is unique & versatile; it has the ability to transform like no other hair. Afro hair is referred to as spongy, woolly, cottony, nappy kinky coily, curly, frizzy. There is no other hair texture like afro hair we are the only people on the planet that have this hair type that makes us unique!

There are many theories as to why black people have this unique hair type. I found some theories listed below that were interesting, poignant and some scientific in their conclusion. The theories below are opinions, you decide if any of these theories resonate with you.

"Afro-textured hair may have initially evolved because of an adaptive need (amongst humanity's hominid ancestors) for protection against the intense UV radiation of Africa. Subsequently (and/or additionally), because the relatively sparse density of Afro-hair, combined with its elastic helix shape, results in an airy effect, the resulting increased circulation of cool air onto the scalp may have served to facilitate our hominid ancestors' body-temperature-regulation while they lived in the open savannah Further, Afro-hair does not respond as easily to moisture/sweat as straight hair. Thus, instead of sticking to the neck and scalp when wet (as do straighter textures), unless totally drenched, it tends to retain its basic springy puffiness. In this sense, in addition to the above-listed causes, the trait may have also been retained/preferred among many equatorial human groups because of its contribution to enhanced comfort levels under warm conditions."
~ Source: Wikipedia

"Genes for Afro-textured or kinky hair has roots near the equator, where sunlight is more prevalent and temperatures are higher. In the same way that darker skin offers UV protection, the coils of kinky hair do the same. Straight hair acts almost as a conductor of UV rays to the scalp. Also, heat and humidity are conducted. In high

temperatures, this can be dangerous to the brain. Kinky hair, however, does not conduct UV rays the same way. In fact, it blocks these rays from the scalp. In addition, the structure of the coils conduct heat AWAY from the scalp and brain (only the top of hair heats up, the airy coils and lower density of kinky hair allow air to come through, keeping the scalp cool.) Also, kinky hair does not respond to sweat and moisture as straight hair does, it is more resistant, eliminating the discomfort of sweaty hair sticking to the neck.Darker skin, kinky hair just makes Black people more able to cope in the hot weather from where they originated. This is why they can withstand heat better than other races."
~ Source: lil_lola

"It's a physiological adaptation to allow African people to dissipate heat quickly and efficiently to prevent sunstroke in the hot climate to which their people are indigenous to."
~ Source: Wiki Answers

"The sun is male and mother earth is female. The sun gives off ether in the form of what is called prominences. The sun has antennae called granulation and Black peoples woolly hair, looks like that granulation. So our woolly hair may correctly be called granulation. If one puts straight strand of hair closer and closer to fire that strand of hair will granulate, it will ball up because of the potency of the heat. Black people carries his and her SUN within. Sun heat genes within the African pygmies were so dense and potent in their bone marrow and reproductive system, they turned the hair kinky, as fire does to straight strand of hair."
~ Source: 'The Nine Ball' Dr Melchisedek Z York

"God designed us that way of course in order to stand the very hot and fierce sun of Africa and other tropical areas, the curlier the hair, or nappy would act as a hat for sun screening. Other nationalities with different environmental variances, such as colder temps with less sun usually have a thinner lighter hair as well as skin color. Have no doubt, God created it all and knew what he was doing."
~ Source: sherfaune

Kissi Kurls

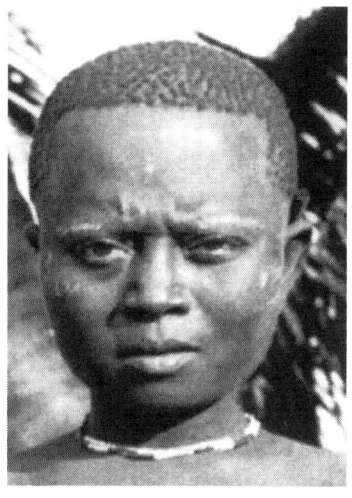

Khoisan (southern Africa)

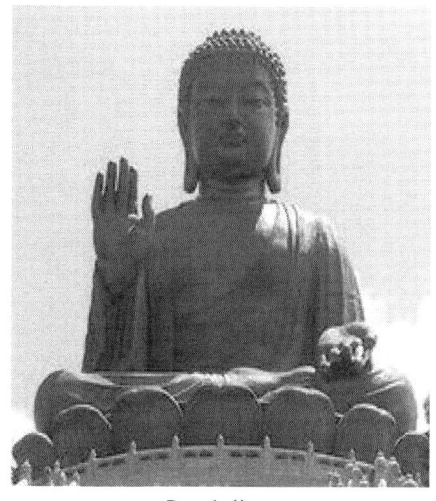

Buddha

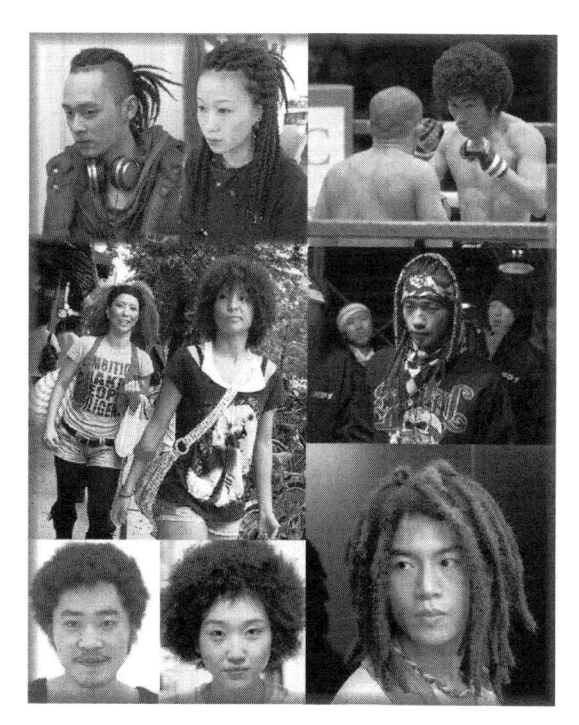

For Years the popular trend in Japan and Korea called the "Afro-perm" or "reggae perm" continues to Grow... "Imitation is the sincerest form of flattery!
Source :'The real Afrikan Truth'

Rocking Your Fro On The Go

Beautiful Big Chop

Referred to by some barbers as the 'number one' in England, and known as the 'Big Chop' in the natural hair world, this short sassy style is for Sistas who want to show the world they ooze confidence and are willing to put their beautiful face out there. This is a Low maintenance hair style, which doesn't mean that you should neglect your hair, on the contrary, to keep this style looking fresh, you will need to moisturize, nourish and hydrate and cut regularly. Accessories with bold beautiful colors that will make you stand out from the crowd.

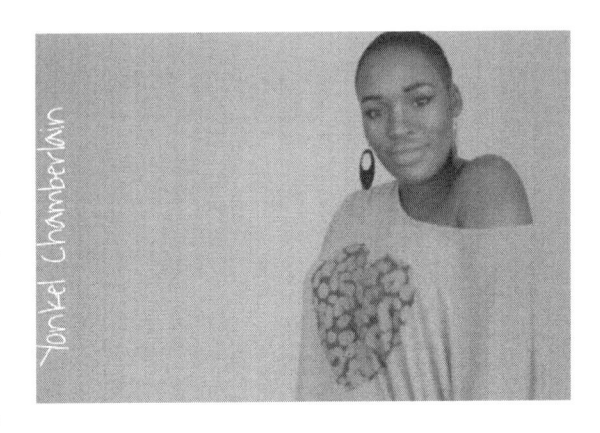

Puff

This classic hair style is great! You can have a low, high or side puff. This style is great for the day or evening, and can be achieved within minutes. You can do jumbo twists for a dramatic effect or small ones to create defined curls. Add an accessory such as a satin headband with detail or a side flower for that summery look.

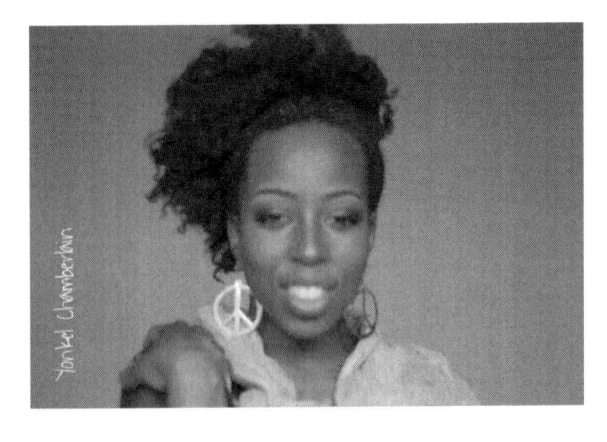

Cornrows/Ghanaian Braids

I love cornrows! One of my favorite styles is the Ghana braids. They differ to cornrows in that to achieve the desired graduated style, you have to use extensions that are gradually added to the hair which initially starts off small and gets wider to your desired width. This low maintenance hair style, is great for girls on the go and want to show off the face. Cornrows cans be styled according to style preference, cornrow ponytails, Mohawk, all back, there are so many creative styles, let your imagination run wild!

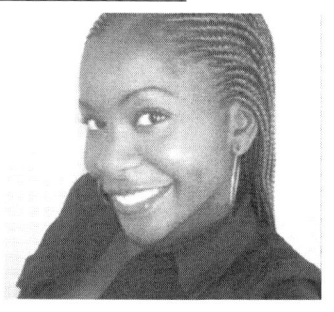

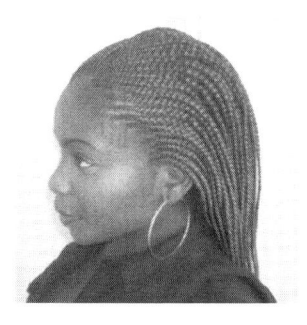

Afro

It's all about big hair, I love hair with volume and the afro is an iconic natural hair style that celebrates liberation, naturalness & unity. Its free flowing signature look embodies cascading curls and various textures, which makes it one of the most loved natural hair styles.

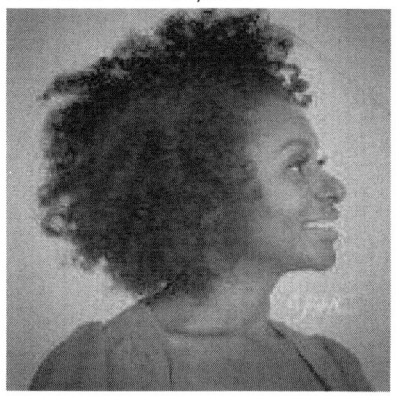

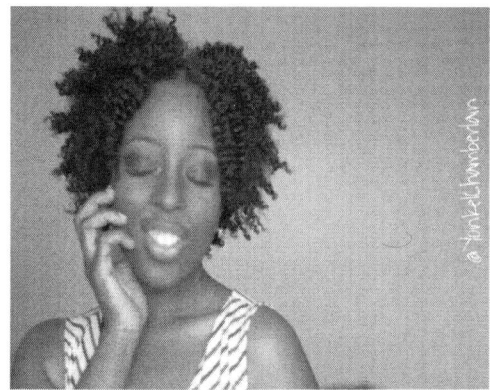

Braids

Braids look so beautiful at any length; this style is on my number one protective style for the winter. This hairstyle allows your tresses to have a break from everyday styling and pulling. Be creative with these beautiful braids change it up with color, size, pick n drop (part braid and left out hair) with so many styling options to choose from this versatile hair style, will keep you looking stylish day in and day out.

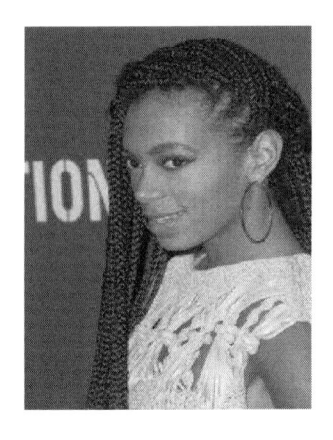

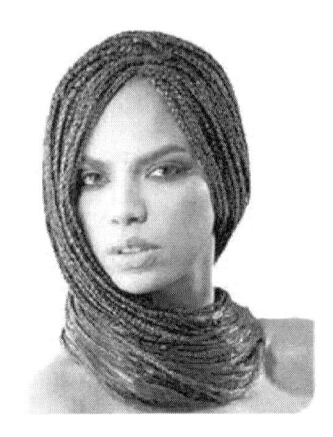

Bantu Knots

The name Bantu means "The People or Humans". Bantu knots are named after the Bantu tribe in Africa that speaks the Bantu language. This traditional African hair style is one of many African hairstyles. This ore inspiring asymmetrical style has presence exposing beautiful features, for those who have defined cheekbones this look is very striking.

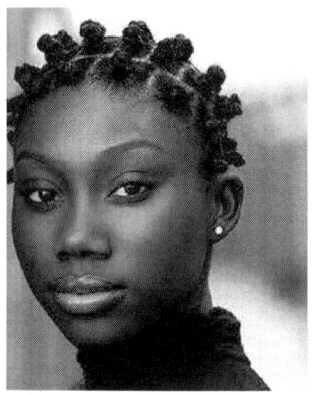

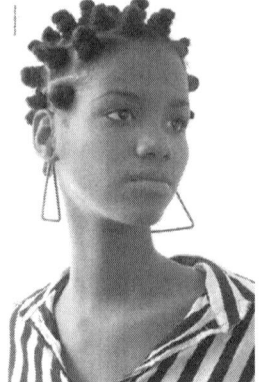

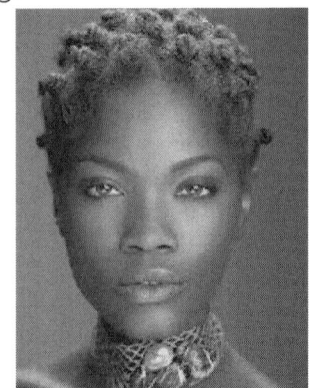

Blow Out

If you're looking for a voluminous hair style with va va voom, minus the flat iron, this hair style is a head turner, a good hairdryer and serum will achieve the perfect blowout.

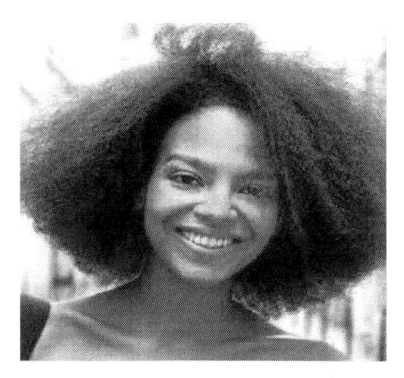

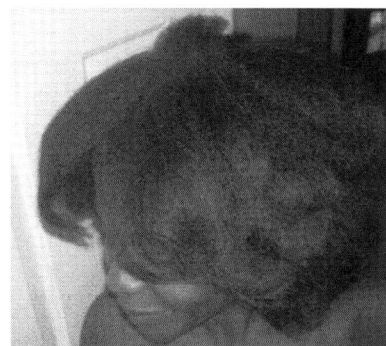

Locks

Locks require time and patience, and contrary to popular belief, this hair style does require maintenance, like most hair styles. There are different types of locks such as sista locks which are very thin locks, free forming- not manipulated, and princess locks that are done with extensions. There are many ways in which to start your locks, comb twist coils, interlocking, two strand twists or braids. At least once a month the new growth can be re-twisted to keep them looking fresh and fabulous.

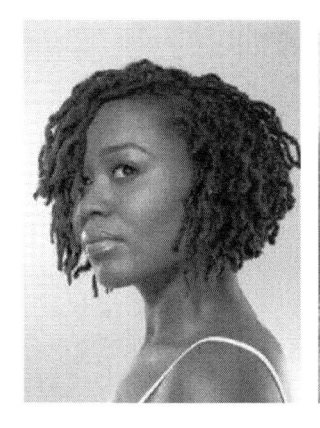

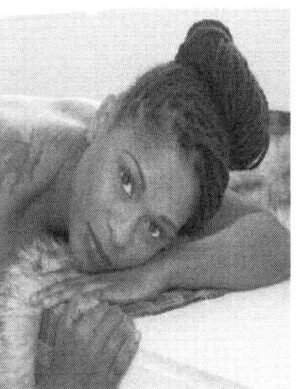

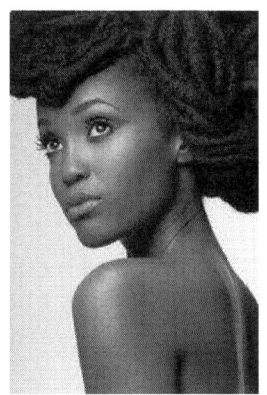

African Threading

I remember having this hair style when I was young, and I can say I appreciate this hair style more as an adult than I did as a child. This hairstyle was commonly done in Ghana and is just one of many artistic African hairstyles, and is on the verge of a huge comeback. This hairstyle is an alternative to blow drying as the thread stretches the hair without the use of heat. This amazing hair style is stunning artistic and trendy. The hair can be threaded wet or dry, It almost takes on a similar look to locks, except threading is easily removed by unraveling the thread and is a temporary style. Once the hair has been threaded unlike locks, it has a more ridged feel although it is very flexible and can be easily bent to create alternative styles. Using different colored threads can bring more attention to this unique style.

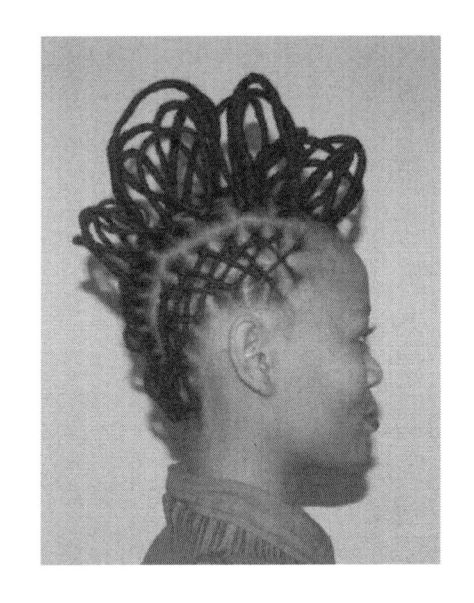

Develop Your Inner Beauty

My definition of inner beauty is a person that displays admirable, humanitarian qualities that consist of compassion, respect, kindness, genuine empathy and care. A person that emits Inner beauty has a natural calmness and peace within them - they are comfortable within their own skin. They reserve their judgment of others, allowing for an interaction and connection so as not to be distracted by outer appearance. They can teach you things that change the way you view the world, they can bring out the best in you, and they are light workers. Workers of light- work for the good of enlightenment and love. I believe inner beauty translates as a glow, a light. This is the basis of the connection that we all can feel when we are amongst them; the light I believe is also a connection to the Most High.

There is too much emphasis on physical beauty. Let's ensure we make time to work on the inner beauty too. It's the inner beauty that will give you that natural beautiful glow.

I feel that there are some beautiful Sistas and Brothers out there, and they do not get the recognition that they deserve for all the good things that they do. If you know of someone out there that you are grateful for, please let them know you appreciate them. It is important to remember those that help us and those that we help, so that we continue to encourage and support those that are less fortunate than ourselves. Do things from the goodness of your heart, not because of money or what reward you hope to receive in return, but because you truly care. I truly believe, that when you do good things, that good things will come back to you.

I felt the need to write this section so as to promote working on one's inner beauty to support the relationships we have with ourselves and others. This is something that needs to be reinforced in our community to strengthen relationships within marriages, between siblings, parents, friends, educators and the authorities. I have provided some exercises that I hope you will find useful. We all have the potential to do well, however, in times of hardship life can become a struggle which can make one become withdrawn, self-centered and sometimes bitter. So I want this to be a reminder that your journey in life is propelled by your determination to overcome obstacles and adversity and, believe me, there is beauty in that.

"There are different kinds of humans, amongst human kind, be a kind human."

Tools Needed
- Notepad
- Pen
- Time

Find a quite place in the house or outside were you want be disturbed. This exercise is a powerful tool to help you discover your inner beauty. Write down all of your good qualities that don't relate to something physical. Are you thoughtful? Loving? Helpful? Positive? All these attributes and a host of others relate to your inner beauty. The process of writing out your strengths gives you tangible evidence of your great inner qualities that you might not have even been aware of. Once you have completed this list, read them out aloud. Ideally you should read this list every day at least for the first six weeks to get into the habit.

Write down one good thing you do or say each day. Show your appreciation to others, and help someone in need. For example, showing appreciation or paying a compliment:
- "*I Love your Natural Hair*"
- "I think you're intelligent"
- "I really appreciate what you have done for me today, thank you"
- "Would you like help with your bags?"
- "I'm going to the shops would you like me to get something for you."

When you wake up each morning, be thankful to see another day, and tell yourself "*I am here for a purpose I am talented, with a wonderful gift to give others.*"

Strengthening Your Inner Beauty

Like Attracts Like
Surround yourself with people that have qualities that you admire, and that will encourage your zest for life, creativity, inspiration and that have your best interests at heart. You are naturally drawn to people that are like you. Be very careful about the company you keep. Observe behaviors and attitudes and if they are not conducive to your well being then distance yourself from such people. These people can hinder your growth. Nobody wants weeds in their garden, so removing them will help you to blossom. Surround yourself with people that possess the qualities you like that will strengthen your inner beauty.

Elders
'*An elder; a person senior in years, who is respected in the Community for their character and spirit, demonstrated through their behavior, good judgment and sensitivity to the*

needs of our community and people. An elder is normally a person of influence in their family and community and is often used to help maintain balance and peace. An elder would include both men and women'.

I did not grow up with my grandparents; I would have enjoyed listening to my grandparent's life journey and their interesting fables and proverbs. I know this because I always try and make time to talk to elders when I'm around them. For instance I recently went to a DIY store and got talking to one of the elders who worked at the store. We conversed for about twenty minutes. During the conversation he told me he had been married for forty years, when I asked him what the factors were that contributed to the longevity of his marriage, he said that when couples come together they must come together for a common goal and that marriage was a training ground. He also went on to say that there was nothing wrong with conflict within a relationship; however the problem today is that people need to remember and understand and have the ability to resolve conflict and a willingness to forgive. He emphasized the importance of being a unit and being an example, not just to your children, but to society. I enjoyed listening to his views and about his journey from the Caribbean to the United States.

It is important to honor our elders and the cultural values that they bring. They are the foundation to ensuring the continuation of traditional African practices and values.

If you are privileged to have your grandparents around, take time out to engage with them, if they are not close by; pick up the phone and call to let them know you are thinking of them. Engaging with a respected elder is good for personal development; it teaches one to listen with the whole self, to be patient, and respectful. They have seen it, done it and been there. Engaging with the elders will aide your personal growth and development, which in turn will strengthen your inner beauty.

Alone Time

In the fast paced world that we live in, we need to remember to make time to gather our thoughts, so that we can recoup from the pressure of life. De-cluttering and freeing your mind so that you are able to effectively function is the reason why it is important to spend time alone. Solitude helps us to develop an inner peace and learn to accept personal space and silence the mind, which is good for relaxation that will help you pay more attention to your inner voice.

Observing Inner Beauty

We all have areas of our life that we can improve. For example, if I see a long queue, I can become quite impatient. My husband told me a story of a person who used to be very impatient and when confronted with a long queue they would rant and rave huff and puff. As queues cannot be avoided and the stress of queuing would make them feel anxious and frustrated, something had to change and it had to be the attitude and mindset. So, one day they decided that they would find the longest queue to join, so that they could learn patience. Any time I show sign of being impatient my husband says this one word 'Saboor' which means patience in Arabic and at that point, I have to check myself and learn to exercise patience. This is a great example of observing our behavior and modifying it so that we can learn to master our weaknesses that in turn may became our strengths. Learn to take care of your inner beauty by reading inspirational and uplifting stories, rewarding yourself for overcoming challenges and loving yourself with all your quirks and flaws. Show compassion, patience, love, and care and practice them daily, with your husband, wife, partner, children, colleagues, neighbors, congregation just about anyone you have regular interaction with. Your inner beauty is unique to you. In practicing this and observing your behavior, you will develop more confidence within yourself and as you become more self assured people will see the confidence within you.

Learn from your mistakes, do not harbor on the past, or regrets. The beauty of the present is we have the opportunity to start a new day with a new way.

Communicate

We must remember that we are in a world with people that have different backgrounds: race, culture, religious views and environments and it is likely that on occasion that you may be misunderstood, or not understand perfectly. In any event, remain respectful especially when trying to communicate difficult feelings.

Try and resolve conflict sooner, rather than later this will help to relieve tension and burden. For, if you are angry or upset, this will manifest and will definitely show and may inhibit your inner beauty.

Creativity

Embark on a new activity that will increase your creativity such as writing poems, painting, woodwork, gardening, writing a journal etc. Creative people invent, imagine, problem-solve, create, and communicate in fresh, new ways. Every business requires creative thinkers in the form of scientists, engineers, medical researchers, technology innovators, business entrepreneurs, artists, performers, writers and illustrators, designers, inventors, educators and parents. Those with the ability to "think outside of the box" will lead the future and make great things happen.

Law Of Attraction

The 'Law of Attraction' if you use it wisely is a very powerful tool. People need to understand that they have the ability to attract good things in their life just by changing their frame of mind. A book called 'The Secret' by author Rhonda Byrne is a good read which talks about the law of attraction. The Secret explains how and why the law of attraction is the most powerful law in the universe. This law governs all energy, attracting like energy to like energy. We are all energy beings, vibrating at a frequency. Depending on what your thoughts, feelings and beliefs are, you will vibrate and emit a certain frequency and likewise you will attract it. Each thought and feeling vibrates on a different frequency. So if you show gratitude, you will emit that frequency and will attract a like energy of gratitude and so on. This is not superstition, or 'spook-ism' this is supported by proven scientific principles.

I have numerous experiences using the law of attraction, when you see the results, it is an amazing feeling, it is now second nature to me. The gist of how it works is, focus on a goal, or desire visualize this goal, with no doubt whatsoever, no thinking of obstacles, how? What? or whens?. With the re-conditioned mind you will see these goals manifest. Adopting this attitude will help strengthen your inner beauty.

Write down the most common terminology you use when speaking about yourself or others.
Do you refer to yourself as stupid, ugly, insignificant, or dumb? Do you speak to or about others the same way? Notice and eradicate defeating vocabulary from yourself talk immediately! Focus on your strengths and if you would like to improve in areas that are weak, as they say 'perfect practice makes perfect'. Replace these words with positive words, I am inventive, I have

a purpose, I am resourceful, I am a mediator, I am smart, I am beautiful etc.

Do the people you associate with more often than not, complain, whine and bitch about their circumstances? People who constantly complain, or always seemed to be involved in conflict, or attract more than often too much negativity in to their life, have no intention of resolving problems or choose not to take action or know how to change their mindset and behavior hence perpetuation a vicious cycle of bad energy.

Take note of how they choose, if they choose, to make an attempt to provide a solution to their problems. Seek positive forward, motivating people.

What questions do you ask about yourself, your life, and your experiences?
Do you use questions that include the words, should" "never" or "always"? Do you ask questions like, "why me what did I do"? Or do you make pronouncements like, "I can't do that!"? Begin right now, to ask questions of yourself that provide solutions instead of blame or wonder. Stop asking the question, "Why?"! Learn to take responsibility and take control of your life.

Take note that what you focus on, does affect your experience and what you focus on the most you will always receive.

The law of attraction does not discriminate, whatever you focus on you will attract. If you say 'I never win anything' the law of attraction will ensure that your wish is granted and lo and behold you will never win anything. Focus on the things you do want. See your thoughts as wishes for what you want in your life. You are able to bring abundance into your life just like the character Aladdin with the genie, think of your thoughts as wishes. Whatever you want you just have to focus, visualize, verbalize, and take action on these desires, and your wish will be granted. If you don't think it will work for you then guess what......it won't work! We are all divine beings that are worthy of abundance & Love you just have to shift your state of mind to knowing that you deserve it!

Embracing Your Curls

Hold a section of hair, look at the intricate curl pattern, and look at the individual strands. Wet a section of the hair and see how the pattern changes form, look at your hair for a couple of minutes and say out aloud what you like about your hair, it must be heartfelt and honest. Here is an example...you must finish with...'I am beautiful' work your way towards each of your body parts from your head to your toes.

"I love my natural hair"
"I love the texture of my hair"
"I love the length of my hair"
"I am grateful that my hair is healthy"
"I like that my hair is so versatile"
"I am beautiful"

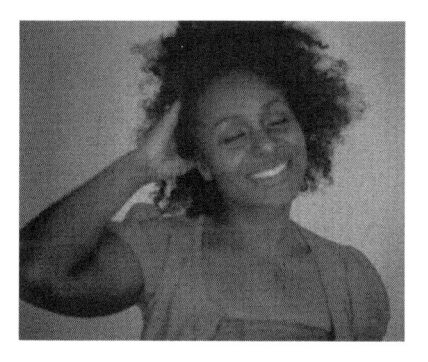

For those that have suffered trauma with their hair, or any part of the body you must remain positive, it is a known fact that thinking positive in times of adversity is critical to your recovery. Think positive thoughts envision what it is you want for yourself and say it with conviction; this will help to manifest your thoughts and dreams into the present.

"Everything has beauty, but not everyone sees it, those who look for beauty, find it"

Hair Psychology - I'm Hair For You

The following exercises are here to help you understand how you truly feel about embarking on your natural hair journey. The idea of this exercise is to look at deep rooted fears or beliefs that could hold you back from moving forward successfully with your hair journey. These questions can also be applied to how you respond to change in general. Writing your feelings down allows you to analyze how you feel and if there is a pattern of behavior. It is a good idea to answers these questions before starting your transition so that you are aware of how you would respond to a bad hair day or a major event.

What damage has the relaxer caused to my hair?

_____
_____
_____
_____
_____
_____
_____
_____

Why do I feel it is important to stop relaxing my hair?

_____
_____
_____
_____
_____
_____
_____

Kissi Kurls

What has inspired me to go natural?

What are my concerns about going natural?

What will I do to understand & manage my natural hair?

How do I respond to change?

Love Your Natural Hair

Does it concern me how other people will react to my natural hair?

Have I tried to go natural in the past? If yes, what will I do differently this time to ensure that I do not revert to putting chemicals on my head?

How many years has it been since I saw my natural hair?

What friends/family/acquaints do I know that have natural hair?
_____
_____
_____
_____
_____
_____
_____
_____

Who are my supporters during this process?
_____
_____
_____
_____
_____
_____
_____
_____
_____

Will having your hair natural affect how you do your job?
_____
_____
_____

Does going to work wearing your hair natural concern You?
_____
_____
_____
_____
_____
_____
_____
_____

Love Your Natural Hair

Will wearing your hair natural impact your job?
_____
_____
_____
_____
_____
_____
_____
_____
_____

Am I emotionally attached to my hair?
_____
_____
_____
_____
_____
_____
_____
_____
_____

What is the current condition of my hair?
_____
_____
_____
_____
_____
_____
_____
_____
_____

Kissi Kurls

What is my bad hair habit (e.g. excessive heat, not conditioning)

___
___
___
___
___
___
___

Is my hair my beauty?

___
___
___
___
___
___

What is the first hair style that I will try when I'm natural?

___
___
___
___
___
___
___

How will I reward Myself when I reach my ultimate goal?

___
___
___
___
___
___

Chapter Five

Interesting Hair Facts

- In West Africa, Ghana and most parts of Africa, the girls and the boys as part of their grooming and presentation have to keep their hair short as low as half an inch. This is practiced so that the girls are not distracted by their hair and keep their focus on their education.

- The word shampoo in English derived from the Hindi word chāmpo and dates back to 1762. The Hindi word referred to head massage usually with hair oil.

- Hair is the second fastest growing tissue in the body; only bone marrow is quicker.

- Women often experience major, but reversible, loss of hair two or three months after giving birth. The massive production of the hormone estrogen during pregnancy puts hair follicles into their 'growth phase'. After the birth, the hormonal balance is restored and the hair follicles go into the 'loss phase', causing a large number of hairs to fall out at once.

- Combing is less detrimental than brushing.

- A developing fetus has all of its hair follicles formed by week 22. At this time there are 5 million follicles on the body. One million of those are on the head, and 100,000 are on the scalp. This is the largest number of follicles we will ever have - follicles are never added during life. As the size of the body increases as we grow older, the density of the hair follicles on the skin decreases.

Love Your Natural Hair

- Madame CJ Walker, commonly known or Sarah Breedlove McWilliams Walker, founded her Hair Care business after suffering from a scalp ailment that caused her to lose some of her hair. Embarrassed by her appearance, she experimented with a variety of home-made remedies and products. She is labeled as the first female black or white woman, to become a self-made millionaire.

- In the north of Africa, Egyptian noblemen and women clipped their hair close to the head. But, for ceremonial occasions, heavy curly-black wigs were donned. Women's wigs were often long and braided, adorned with gold ornaments or ivory hairpins. Men's faces were generally clean shaved, but stiff false beards were sometimes worn.

- There are three types of hair: terminal, villus, and lanugo. Terminal hair is the fully developed, thick, coarse hair found on the head, underarms, and pubic area of a human. Villus hair is the short, very fine hair that covers almost every part of the human body except the palms of the hands, soles of the feet, back of the ears, certain external genital organs, and the lips. Lanugo hair is the hair that covers a fetus, and is also sometimes found on anorexics to help their malnourished bodies retain heat.

- The only part of the hair that is alive is the root where new hair grows. The rest of the hair shaft is made up entirely of dead cells called keratin, which is a type of protein made up of long chains of amino acids.

- Due to the many tribal customs, African hairstyles were many and varied and usually signified status. Maasai warriors tied the front hair into sections of tiny braids whilst the back hair was allowed to grow to waist length. Non-warriors and women however shaved their heads. Many tribes dyed the hair with red earth and grease – some even stiffened it with animal dung. The complex style of the Mangbetu women involved braiding the hair thinly and arranging over a cone-shaped basket frame, flaring the top then adorning the whole thing with long, bone needles. Other tribes such as the Miango took a more simple approach, covering their long ponytails with a headscarf and adorning with leaves.

- Hair grows an average of half an inch per month with growth being predetermined by a person's genetic code. In a year, hair can grow up to 6 inches. As a person ages, hair growth can slow to about one-quarter inch per month. New hair cells form in the root as the hair cells divide, and push the hair forward, making it longer. The new hair is always added at the root as the older hair inches downward. Hair grows at the same rate on every part of the head. Even though hair growth is determined by genes, hormones released in the body during the summer season can increase the rate of growth. However, the growth rate is relatively small--about 0.05 inches more than on average. Thus, hair does actually grow a little bit faster in the summer.

- Darker Hair contains higher levels of melanin than blonde hair; darker hair therefore protects you from the sun. Also darker colors absorbs more sunlight than lighter colors, thus darker hair enables you to receive an abundance of vitamin D.

- Afro hair grows up towards the sun, and in some ancient depictions of Kings and Queens this is regarded as a crown.

- It is normal to lose about 100 hairs per day from your scalp.

- Although archaeologists have used the name "Olmec," to refer to the Black builders of ancient Mexico's first civilizations, recent discoveries have proven that these Olmecs were West Africans. Hairstyles such as Cornrows are found on many of the Afro-Olmec terracotta found in Mexico, and in parts of the world such on paintings statues and figurines. Both kinky hair carved into one of the colossal stone heads of basalt, as well as the Cornrowed style wearing tassels. The "Cornrow" factor clearly shows that Africans in Mexico in prehistoric times most likely came from the West Africa/South Sahara region, rather than Melanesia. It is in West Africa that Cornrows are very common and have been since prehistoric times.

- 90% of scalp hairs are growing while the 10% of hair are resting.

- Female hair grows a lot slower than male hair, not a significant amount about 0.075mm a month. The increased hair growth in males is due to testosterone, which produces faster growth and longer hair.

- The removal of unwanted body hair can be dated back to the time of the ancient Egyptians, who used abrasion as a way to remove hair. Ancient Romans and Greeks used pumice stones and other abrasives to remove hair. Native Americans and Pacific Islanders removed hair by scraping with seashells. In ancient Mayan and Aztec cultures, the volcanic glass obsidian was used to shave hair. Obsidian can be honed many times sharper than most razor blades. The glassy material comes in a range of colors from black to green to bright orange, and it is found everywhere rhyolite-rich volcanic deposits are found.

- The Maasai tribe of Kenya are great warriors, one of deep culture and strict tradition; they are the most famous tribe of

Kenya. They are also known for their intricate hairstyles. These styles are only worn by the Maasai warrior men. They spend hours braiding each other's hair, the result are micro braids equally sized. The reddish color of their hair comes from clay and red ochre. Red ochre is a natural earth pigment found around volcanic regions. The Maasai mix the ochre with animal fat to get a grease paint consistency and then apply it to their hair. This grease paint dries quickly and covers surfaces thoroughly. They paint their hair without using toxic dyes, and they also have very elaborate brightly colored headdresses.

- The average life span of a strand of hair is about 4-7 years.

- Clay locs: The Himba tribe lives in the mountainous regions of Kaokoland in Namibia. Himba's are nomad's, moving with their cattle as the times change. Despite their constant moving, the Himba women keep their routine going. Part of the Himba woman's tradition is to spend several hours a day dedicated to their beauty. The Himba women smear their skin twice a day with a paste called Otjize, which is a mixture of rancid butter, ash and ochre, it serves as perfume and protects them from the desert climate the same paste they use in their hair to make their intricate hairstyles. Otijize is not the only thing Himba women put in their hair, they use the hair of their family members to make their braids appear longer. Their hair is redone every three months and can take up to 2 days. Similar to other cultures around the world the hair of the Himba women is very symbolic. In the Himba tribe you can tell a woman's marital status by her hair as well as her maturity. Little girls usually wear braids until they reach puberty. Once a girl has hit puberty she is kept in doors for five days. While in doors a goat is slaughtered in their honor and its skin is used to make the centre piece of her headdress as seen in the pictures.

Love Your Natural Hair

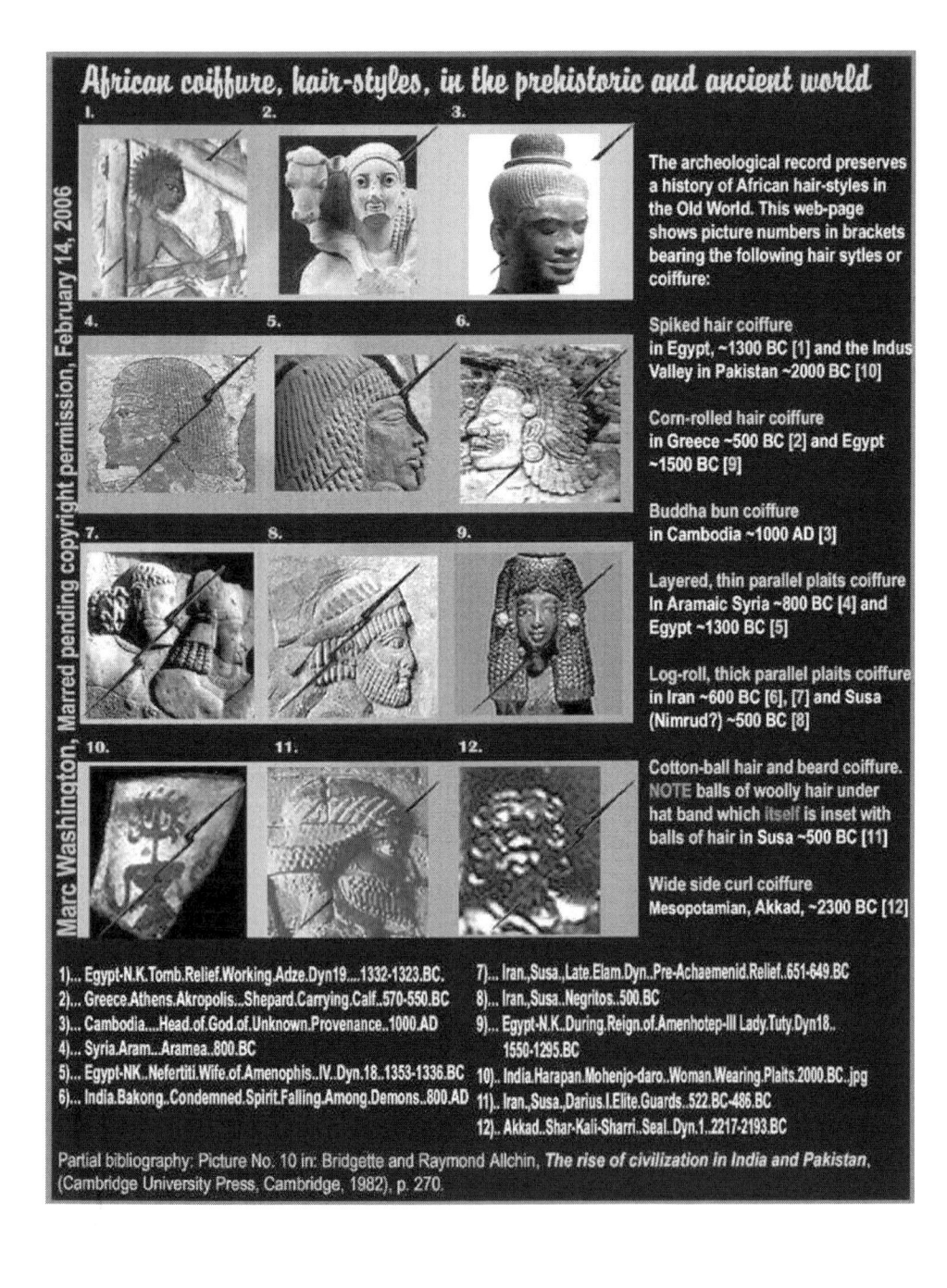

African coiffure, hair-styles, in the prehistoric and ancient world

Marc Washington, Marred pending copyright permission, February 14, 2006

The archeological record preserves a history of African hair-styles in the Old World. This web-page shows picture numbers in brackets bearing the following hair sytles or coiffure:

Spiked hair coiffure
in Egypt, ~1300 BC [1] and the Indus Valley in Pakistan ~2000 BC [10]

Corn-rolled hair coiffure
in Greece ~500 BC [2] and Egypt ~1500 BC [9]

Buddha bun coiffure
in Cambodia ~1000 AD [3]

Layered, thin parallel plaits coiffure
in Aramaic Syria ~800 BC [4] and Egypt ~1300 BC [5]

Log-roll, thick parallel plaits coiffure
in Iran ~600 BC [6], [7] and Susa (Nimrud?) ~500 BC [8]

Cotton-ball hair and beard coiffure.
NOTE balls of woolly hair under hat band which itself is inset with balls of hair in Susa ~500 BC [11]

Wide side curl coiffure
Mesopotamian, Akkad, ~2300 BC [12]

1)... Egypt-N.K.Tomb.Relief.Working.Adze.Dyn19....1332-1323.BC.
2)... Greece.Athens.Akropolis...Shepard.Carrying.Calf..570-550.BC
3)... Cambodia....Head.of.God.of.Unknown.Provenance..1000.AD
4)... Syria.Aram...Aramea..800.BC
5)... Egypt-NK..Nefertiti.Wife.of.Amenophis..IV..Dyn.18..1353-1336.BC
6)... India.Bakong..Condemned.Spirit.Falling.Among.Demons..800.AD
7)... Iran.,Susa.,Late.Elam.Dyn..Pre-Achaemenid.Relief..651-649.BC
8)... Iran.,Susa..Negritos..500.BC
9)... Egypt-N.K..During.Reign.of.Amenhotep-III Lady.Tuty.Dyn18.. 1550-1295.BC
10).. India.Harapan.Mohenjo-daro..Woman.Wearing.Plaits.2000.BC..jpg
11).. Iran.,Susa.,Darius.I.Elite.Guards..522.BC-486.BC
12).. Akkad..Shar-Kali-Sharri..Seal..Dyn.1..2217-2193.BC

Partial bibliography: Picture No. 10 in: Bridgette and Raymond Allchin, *The rise of civilization in India and Pakistan*, (Cambridge University Press, Cambridge, 1982), p. 270.

Kissi Kurls

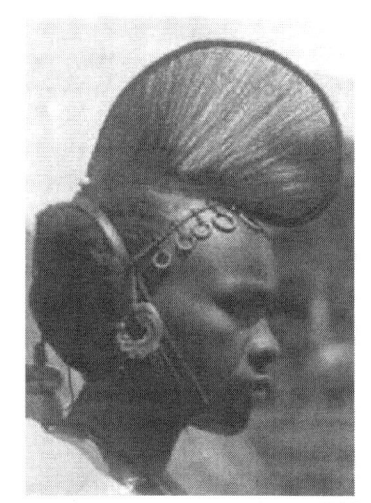

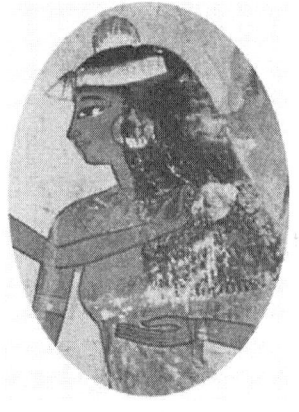

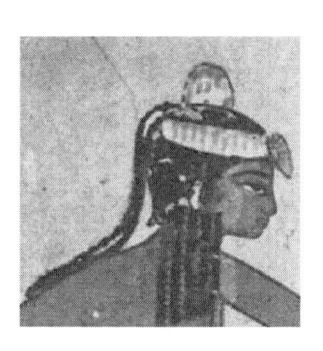

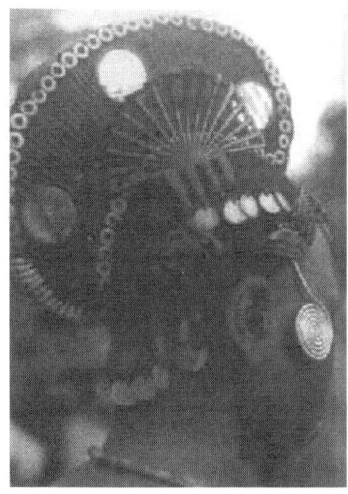

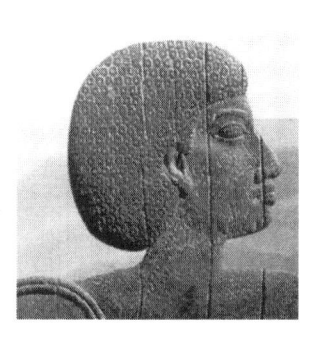

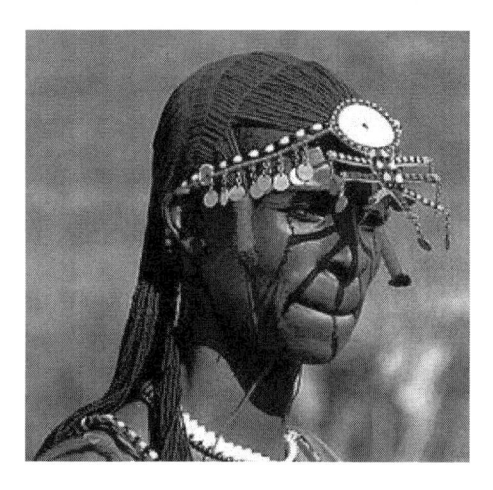

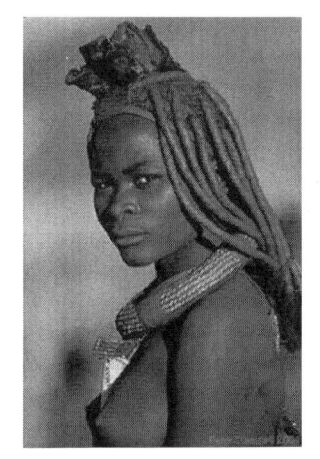

Love Your Natural Hair

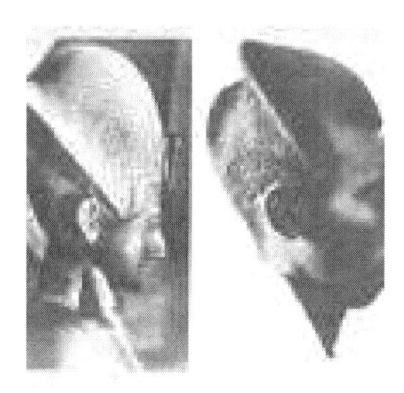

War Crown (above & left) and this Watusi hairstyle (right). You can see the similarities between the two hair styles. The significance of the coils depicted in the Egyptian War crown are representative of the tight curl pattern of Afro hair. Many of the hair styles above are still prevalent hair styles today.

- The word "Cosmos" meaning order or "Ma,at" an ancient Egyptian deity that represents truth, justice, harmony, balance, order, Reciprocity, Propriety, can also be found in the word "Cosmetology". The word cosmetology literally means 'to arrange or put in order' (to perform Ma'at) but is used to refer to the science and art of beautification which includes hairstyling, skin care, manicures, pedicures, cosmetics ect. Cosmetology, applying Ma'at as the science and art of beautification is an art that African women have been doing for thousands of years. The mathematical process of applying Ma'at, order and arrangement for beautification (cosmetology in modern language) involves creating symmetrical geometric patterns that are aesthetically pleasing, proportional and balanced.

- It has been scientifically shown that geometric facial symmetry is a trait that humans find most attractive and desirable, therefore one of the goals of applying Ma'at in Cosmetology is to make the face appear symmetrical the results of this is beautification, attraction, and procreation.

Kissi Kurls

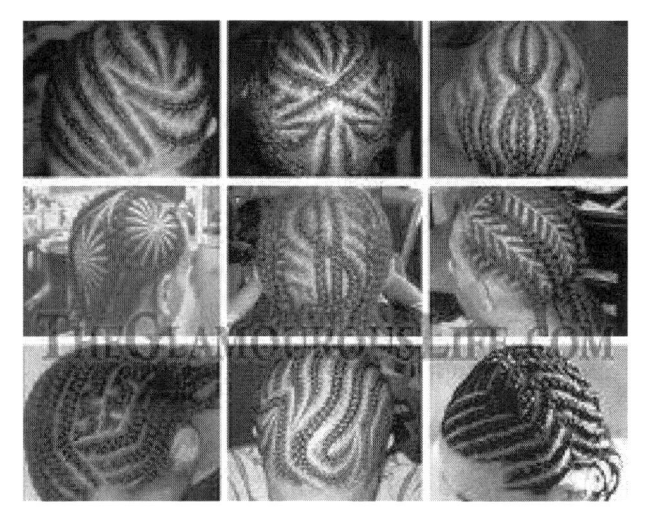

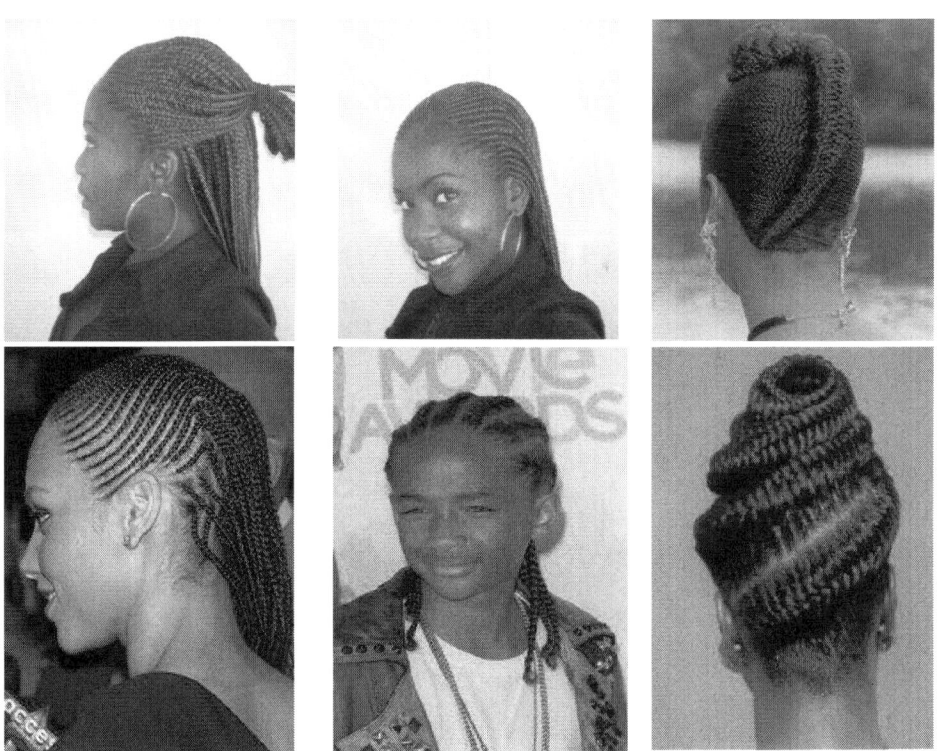

Traditional African hair styles are symmetrical and geometric which all relate to mathematics.

Dead or Alive?

There is some controversy as to whether hair is actually dead or alive. In my opinion, I subscribe to the idea that hair has a source of life, though the hair itself is not 'alive', it's connected to life. Hair is described as dead because the strands of hair outside of your scalp are physiologically dead, it has no blood, nerves or muscles, when you cut it there is no pain, and it undergoes no further destructive (catabolic) change. However, it is connected to life! For a dead fiber, it is quite remarkable. Healthy hair can be stretched up to 30% of its length; can absorb its own weight in water and can increase its diameter by 20%.

Hair can be colored, shaped, texturized; we can wash it, brush it, set it, pull it and rub it to an amazing degree and yet despite all of this, our hair can remain resilient and durable! When hair is connected to a living being, it has a source of life that feeds its growth and ensures its survival. If hair falls out or if you pluck out hair strands at the scalp, then hair has been removed from the living source that feeds and nurtures its continuity. The strand of hair cannot continue to grow without its source; therefore it can be officially described as dead. Just like a leaf that has left a plant.

In my opinion hair has energetic properties when it's on your head, and is dead when removed from the root. I say my hair is *alive*. Hair that looks this good and is so versatile, in my opinion, is surely not *dead*.

Kissi Kurls

Natural Afro hair when combed out also serves as shade from the sun. You can see yourself in nature too.

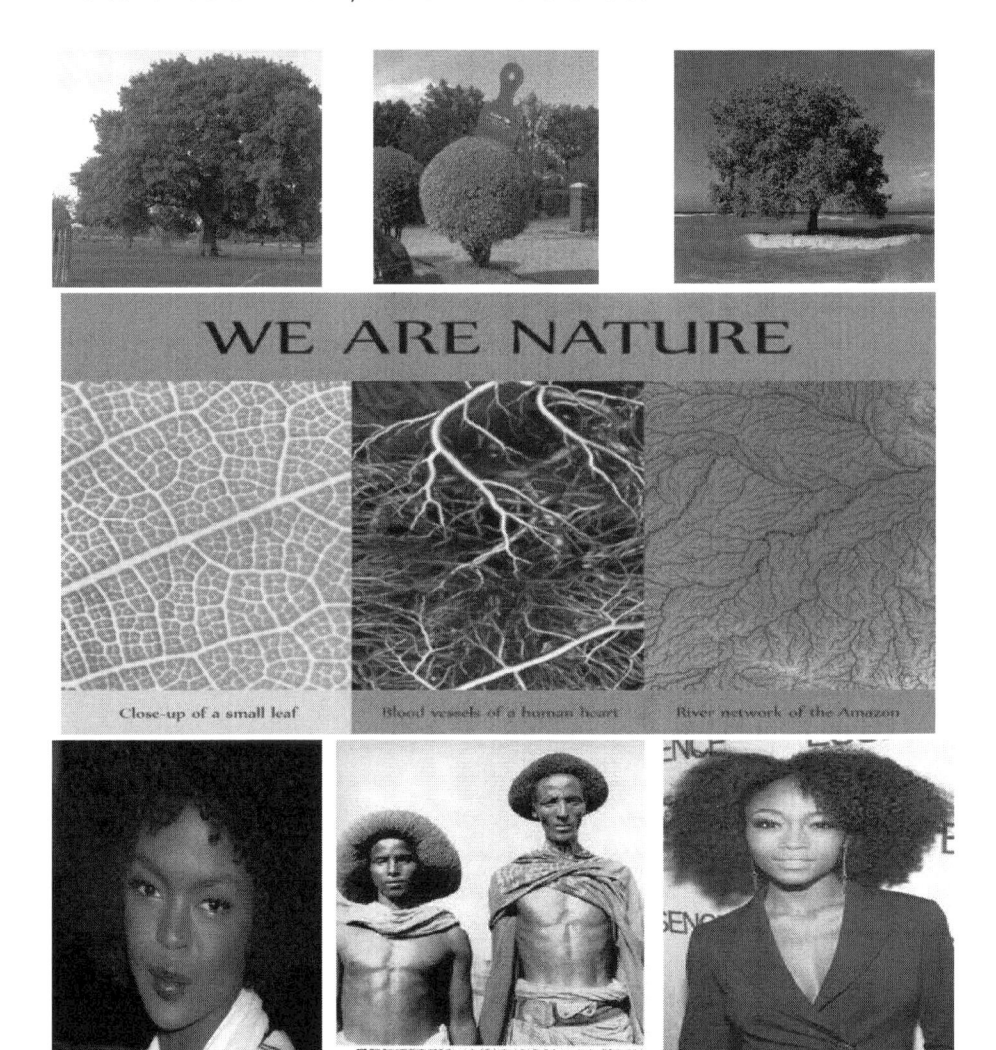

WE ARE NATURE

Close-up of a small leaf   Blood vessels of a human heart   River network of the Amazon

www.KissiKurls.com 187

African Combs

In this section we are going to look at the historical and modern day uses of African, ancient Egyptian combs and how our ancestors used these combs and their significance at that time.

A comb is usually described as a flat, solid tool with teeth. The etymology of the word comb goes back to ancient Greek or Sanskrit meaning 'to bite, tooth, and molar tooth'. The definition of a comb as stated in Wikipedia is: 'a toothed device used in hair care for straightening and cleaning hair or other fibers'. So according to Wikipedia's definition, everyone that combs their hair, also wants to straighten it? No, sorry Wikipedia; I comb my hair to detangle it, not everyone is trying to conform to having straight hair. So be mindful of subliminal wording, adverts, slogans or messages, they don't always get it right!

Combs are among the oldest human tools found by archaeologists, when excavating in areas such as Africa. Africa is the richest continent on earth for natural resources and history.

Today's Combs are commonly made from plastic as it is cheaper and faster to manufacture, however, other materials, are used to make combs, such as metal, bone or wood. Ivory and tortoiseshell were once common but concerns for the animals that produce them have reduced their usage. When made from wood, combs are largely made of boxwood cherry wood or other fine-grained woods. Good quality, wooden combs are usually handmade and polished. Nowadays, specialists advocate the use of wide-toothed, wooden combs in place of hairbrushes and fine-toothed plastic combs. Wooden hair combs are anti static and have no sharp seams, and therefore are unlikely to snap or tangle the hair further. It is said that combing the hair has an acupuncture-like effect. The cranial nerves become stimulated during the process. Holistic medicine practitioners strongly advise the use of combs to aid in getting over a feeling of depression. To return to a feeling of well being, with a bounce, use gentle stokes to caress the scalp, building up a rhythmic action all over the head. It is not necessary to comb through the hair, just massage the scalp with the teeth of the comb or alternatively you can also use your finger and massage the scalp with some essential oils to invigorate and revitalize yourself and your hair.

Whilst doing my research on this subject I came across a lot of articles comparing and contrasting wooden combs to plastic combs, and the pros and cons of both. Up until this point I had been using plastic combs on my own hair, I then made a conscious decision to switch to wooden combs. I feel that natural material products and tools personally resonate with me and the journey that I'm on, which is to be in tune with nature by using organic products that can be found or sourced locally or within our environment, or by recycling, thus being environmentally friendly. You can make a choice of what material to use as it is for you to decide what you prefer.

Some women report that they did not see the difference between the two different materials whilst other reports suggest that there is a significant difference for them when they switched from plastic to wooden combs and they wouldn't go back. Here are some of the reported benefits:

Love Your Natural Hair

These are the statistics from a poll:

I've used a wooden comb and it makes a huge difference	38.11%
I've used a wooden comb and didn't see a difference	13.83%
I haven't tried one, but want to	44.42%
Wooden combs are a scam	3.64%

Benefits
- Described as luxurious
- Anti bacterial
- Smooth glide
- Less breakage
- Helps simulate circulation
- Eliminates static
- Helps to distribute the oils in the hair more easily
- Clean only with oils not water
- Last a lifetime

Petrie Museum

Flinders Petrie was an English Egyptologist and a pioneer of systematic methodology in archaeology and the preservation of artifacts unearthed. Flinders Petrie was the founder of the Petrie Museum based in London England. The Petrie Museum houses an estimated 80,000 objects, making it one of the greatest collections of African Egyptian and Sudanese archaeology in the world. Some ancient hair tools are on display at the Petrie Museum which is open to the public. The museum has also held a workshop on African combs. I decided, therefore, to go to the Petrie Museum to interview Dr Sally-Ann Ashton, and find out more about these ancient

Egyptian artifacts and the importance and relevance of these fascinating and beautiful tools that adorned the heads of the world's greatest Emperors and Empresses.

Hair grooming has always played an important role in the culture of Africa and the African Diaspora and the traditional African comb, know as an African pick, rake or Afro' has played a crucial role in the creation, maintenance, and decoration of hair-styles. The comb is used by both men and women, and continues to be relevant to both groups in the present day.

I was intrigued and excited about the revelations, mysteries, cultures and traditions of African Egyptian combs. When I arrived, I was greeted by Dr Sally-Ann Ashton, a researcher in Ancient Egypt and Sudan. The seminar had a good number of attendees. We were about to go on a journey in time and gain insight and knowledge about our ancestors. We would make connections between the past and the present ways of looking after our hair.

What I thought especially admirable are Dr Sally Ann Ashton's motivations and goals, which are to strengthen the arguments connecting Ancient Egypt to traditional African origins and culture. She expressed the idea that there is a tendency of some of the other Egyptologists to try and isolate African Egyptian hair care from that of the continent.

During the seminar Dr Sally-Ann Ashton highlighted many of the links between ancient depictions of hair and traditional ones, as well as relationships between modern Afro hair styling techniques and practices and ancient; with braids being just one example of many.

We were shown slides of African Egyptians who were buried with combs in their hair and others with combs wrapped in hair beside them. Also, in some places, it would have been impossible to buy a comb from anyone other than a specialist and combs, if made by women, would first have to be cleansed before they could be sold.

We were also shown quotes by the museum's founder Petrie, who stated that he had observed notable differences between hair combs used by ancient Egyptians and those in use by Europeans. Dr Sally-Ann Ashton has been exploring what this could show us in more depth and admitted that much of her time recently has been spent measuring the distance between the teeth of various ancient combs which may provide very important evidence, regarding the origin, and previously dominant, African presence in Egypt.

She also revealed that the increased European presence in Egypt corresponds with the gradual narrowing of the distance between comb teeth. In addition to this, she explained that prior to the increased European presence in Africa, many of the combs were carved with images and motifs which represented animals and often gods, but this common practice declined (for example, with Roman influence) and thus everyday references to traditional Gods was reduced. Instead these appear to have been replaced with standardized patterns. I found the workshop to be very informative, revealing, and interesting. Here are some of the combs exhibited in the Petrie museum.

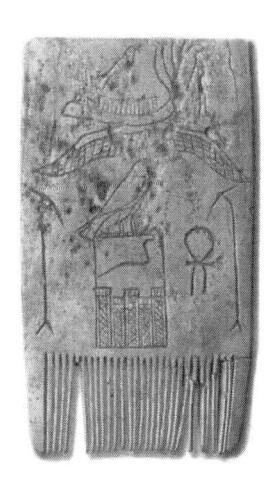

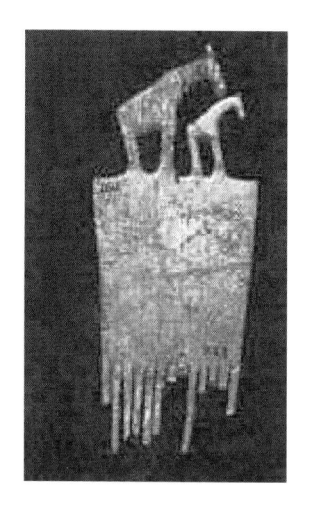

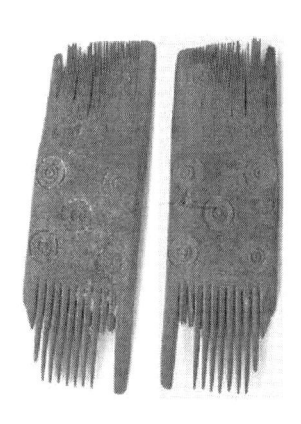

In the twentieth century 'afro' combs have taken on a wider political and cultural message, perhaps most notably in the form of the 'Black Fist' comb that references the Black power salute.

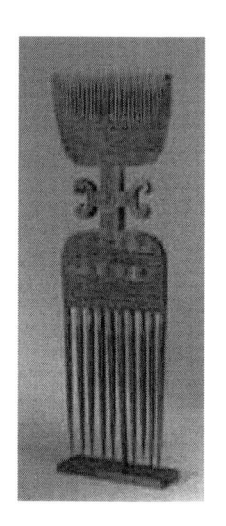

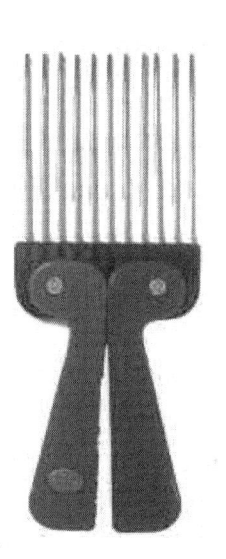

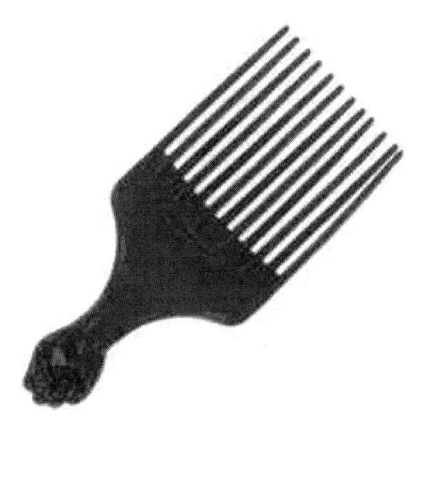

Interesting Comb Facts

The Kazoo's distant relative is the "Mirliton," which goes back centuries in Africa. It was made in a variety of shapes and sizes from natural materials such as bone, gourds, bark and animal horns. Kazoo instruments have been used in Africa for hundreds of years, to disguise their voices, or to imitate animals, often for various ceremonial purposes. According to legend, it was on such an instrument that the kazoo, invented in the 19th century by an African American named Alabama Vest in Macon, Georgia, United States, is based. To date it is estimated that tens of millions of kazoos have been sold in the U.S. alone. Some have called the kazoo a toy but the truth is that professional musicians in all genres, from jazz to classical, have used the Kazoo in their arrangements and recordings. Today you can see people on 'Youtube' using a modern comb shown in the picture below in fig 1, which can be also used as a musical instrument. To get the sound you have to wrap either a piece of plastic like a plastic bag, leaf or paper over the comb, and humming on it with cropped lips produce a heavenly ethereal sound. This principle is used in a musical instrument called the Kazoo shown below in fig 2. The shape, material and length of the teeth determine the harmonic qualities of the comb.

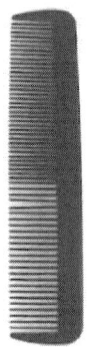

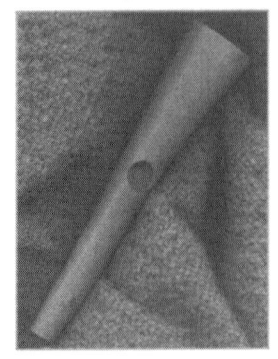

fig1   fig2 An African' Mirliton'(Kazoo) made from a gourd

- A used comb, will hold a person's DNA, this is the first item that police investigators will seek on a crime scene as the remaining hair dandruff left in the comb will give clues as to whether to prove or disprove an accusation.

- Many African prints such as the African cloths in Ghana depict the symbol of an afro comb. The combs symbolize fertility and beauty which is also associated with the deity Hathor, the fertility goddess who leads women into the afterlife.

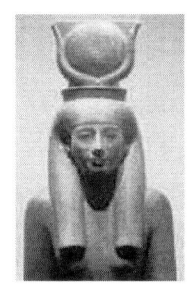

Hathor Deity-fertility & beauty

- Among Hindus, during the period of mourning the family is not supposed to brush, comb or oil the hair. For some groups this continues for a fortnight. After the last rites, the men shave off their hair while the women have the not so pleasant task of combing the tangled mass.

- There is an official club called the Antique Comb Collectors Club a non-profit organization that was founded in 1985, when three like minded ladies from different regions of the country started with a newsletter. Since its inception it now has members located in the US, Canada, England, France, the Netherlands and Switzerland. The ACCCI is composed of novice experts who share an interest in vintage ornaments for the hair. http://www.antiquecombclub.com

Comb (Kanga) – CLEANLINESS

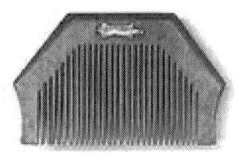

- In Sikh religion, the kanga is similar to a small comb and affirms its bearer's commitment to society. It is tucked neatly in a Sikh's uncut hair. Just as a comb helps to remove the tangles and cleans the hair, the Kanga is a spiritual reminder to shed impurities of thought.

- The Egyptians worried about hair loss as other people have done throughout history. A hair restorer made for Queen Shesh mother of King Teti was concocted by boiling up the hoof of an ass, the stone of a date and the paw of a female greyhound. This ointment was applied liberally throughout the hair.

- The Ancient African Egyptians women adorned their wigs with tassels, tiara, beads using pins and combs to hold the curls in place.

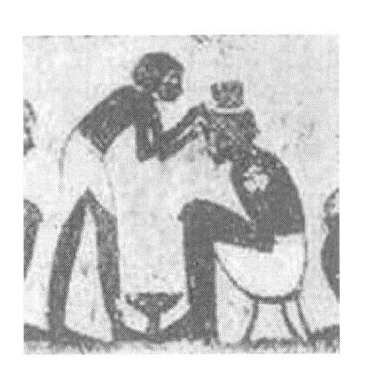

Barber shaving the head of a soldier
Tomb of Userhat, 18th dynasty
Source: V. Easy

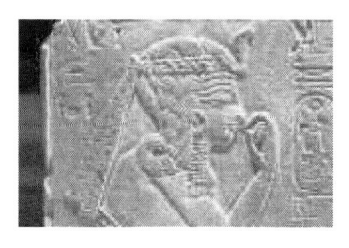

Royal child with side lock
New Kingdom
Source: Jon Bodsworth

Grey Hair

Grey hair was hidden by the application of henna since the middle of the 4th millennium BCE at least. Sometimes it was tinted with an ointment containing the astringent juniper-berries and two other, unidentified plants which supplied the coloring agent. But magic was also tried: blood of a black ox, the ground black horn of a gazelle or putrid donkey's liver were hoped to prevent greying .One should think that in a society where people often had clean shaved heads baldness would not be much of a problem, but it seems some disliked losing their hair and combated it by applying oils and fats or placing chopped lettuce leaves on their skin.

Ken & Barbie? How about Ama & Kojo

When I was growing up black dolls were scarce, you would have more chance of finding a needle in a hay stack than finding a black doll in a toy store. However, I am noticing the presence of black dolls in more shops now than before, although there is not much choice. They tend to have straight hair and European features. The dolls in the shops tend to be limited. Black dolls should be a reflection of the diversity of black children ranging from skin complexion, hair textures and styles.

Within our community if there are services or products that do not cater to us then we should invent and create the product to satisfy the demands that meet our needs.

I realized how challenging finding a doll with natural hair was going to be when I wanted to have a natural hair doll for my wedding. I stumbled across Karen Bryd creator of 'Natural Girls United' and I was relieved and in high spirits to see artistic, creative natural hair styles and the various brown hues ranging from almond complexion to deepest darkest velvet chocolate skin, and stylishly trendy clothes that embody the beautiful black dolls. I absolutely love the collection of dolls and so does every child that visits us in our home. The children tend to gravitate towards them, wanting to play with the dolls. The children appear to be curious and feel a sense of familiarity and comfort seeing dolls that have their natural hair texture finally on a doll.

Karen Byrd: "*I have wanted to take-on the project of customizing dolls hair, to have the look and feel of styles and textures of African American & Mulit-Cultural (ethnic) women and girls, for a long time. As a young girl, I remember loving to play with my dolls... mainly with my Barbie dolls. I thought the dolls where beautiful, but always noticed that my African American dolls did not look like me. Their features did* not look like mine and their hair certainly did not look or feel like mine! This did affect my view of what beauty was. In articles, videos and news stories such as Black Girls Want White Dolls, What a Doll Tells Us About Race, Black Doll White Doll, White and black children biased toward lighter skin & A Girl Like Me - it is apparent that this is something that affects many children and adults; and that there is a need for positive community change.

The Natural Girls United! project has turned into a business, and is something that I hope will help to bring a positive view of what ethnic beauty is. There is a serious need for our young girls to be able to have dolls that look like them. It is something that affects their self esteem and confidence, and how they view themselves. There have been quite a few studies done that show that African American boys and girls often think of black dolls as bad and white dolls as good. Of course, this is not something that the parent is teaching their child. So why are they getting these mixed messages about good and bad skin color, or good and bad hair? It all has to do with the images they see as they grow up.

If a child is constantly looking at images, dolls, television, books and magazines - and only seeing beauty as something or someone with non-ethnic features and long, straight hair - then they are going to assume that this is what beauty is. It is something that has hurt our young people for centuries. But each day we learn that it is important to show them and teach them that their beauty is beautiful."

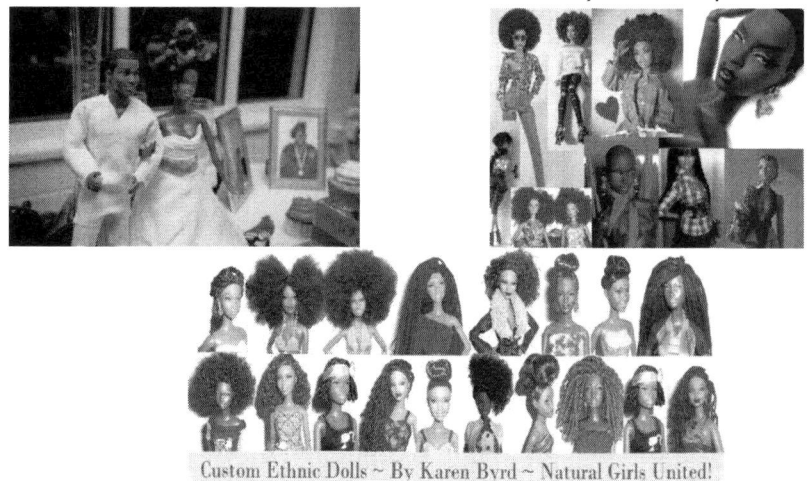

Custom Ethnic Dolls ~ By Karen Byrd ~ Natural Girls United!

Natural Girls United-Karen Byrd www.naturalgirlsunited.com

Love Your Natural Hair

The Clark experiment, also known as the 'The Black & White dolls experiment', was conducted by Psychologist Dr Kenneth Clark and his wife, psychologist Dr Mamie Phipps Clark. The children were given black and white dolls to play with, and asked to indicate which doll they would prefer to play with. The results showed that regardless of community, black children identified with the black dolls, but that children of both races tended to view the white dolls favorably and the black dolls unfavorably, as playthings. Clark's results were published in a 1950 paper, "Effects of Prejudice and Discrimination on Personality Development," in which he concluded that institutional discrimination, including racial segregation in public schools, was harmful to the personality and psychological development of black children.

In August 2012, I conducted an experiment called the Natural Hair Doll Test. This experiment took place at a Natural Hair event. The children's ages ranged from 3 - 9 years old, they were shown a black doll with kinky hair and a white doll with straight hair. The children had to choose between them which doll they preferred. The majority of the children in the experiment leaned more towards the doll with the natural hair, embracing the strands of the dolls hair and playing with it during the interview not shying away from it, as if it was foreign but familiar.

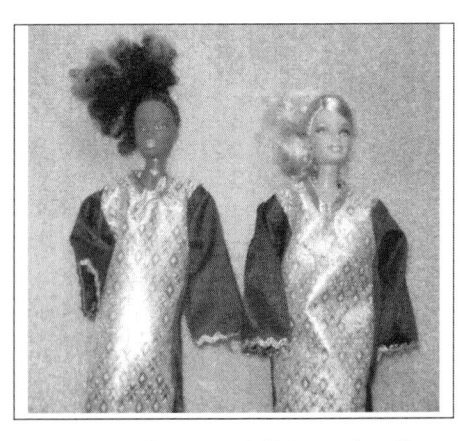

- The age range of the children who participated in the Natural Hair Doll experiment ranged from age 3 to age 9.
- 20% of the participants were male and 80% of the participants were female.

Kissi Kurls

The questions asked during the Natural Hair Doll experiment were:

1. Which doll is the pretty doll?
2. Why is the doll pretty?
3. Which doll is the Ugly doll?
4. Why is the doll Ugly?
5. Which doll had good hair?
6. Why is the hair good?
7. Which doll has bad hair?
8. Why is the hair bad?
9. Which doll is the nice doll?
10. Why is that the nice doll?
11. Which doll is the bad doll?
12. Why is that the bad doll?
13. Point to the doll that looks most like you.

The results of the Natural Hair Doll experiment were:

Which doll is the pretty doll?

- BLACK DOLL: 80%
- WHITE DOLL: 20%

www.KissiKurls.com

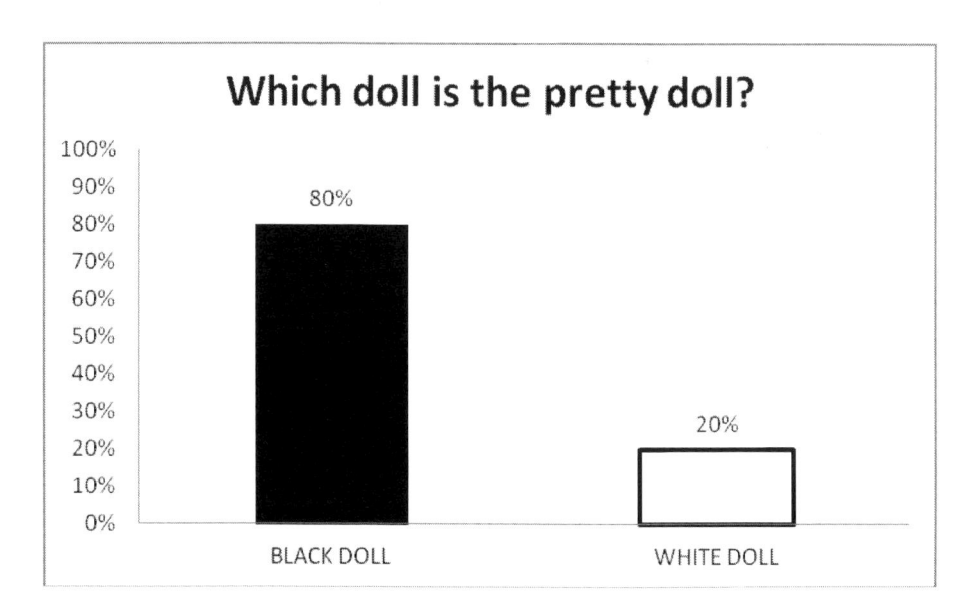

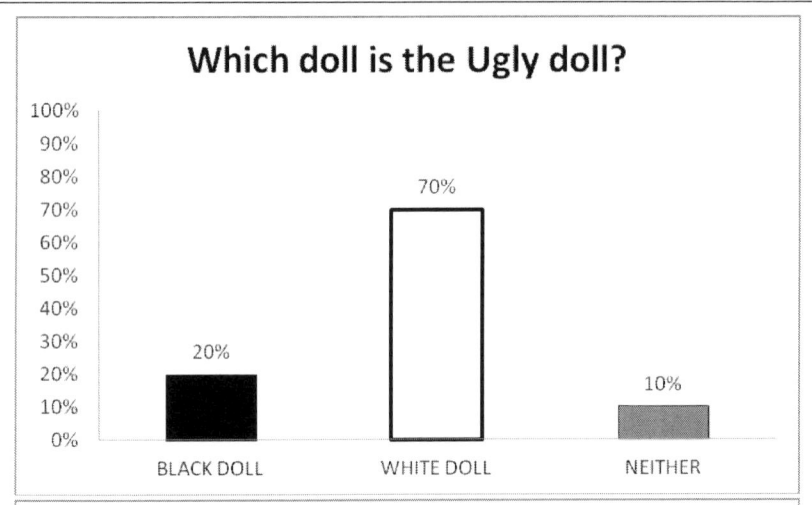

Love Your Natural Hair

Which doll is the Ugly doll?

- BLACK DOLL: 20%
- WHITE DOLL: 70%
- NEITHER: 10%

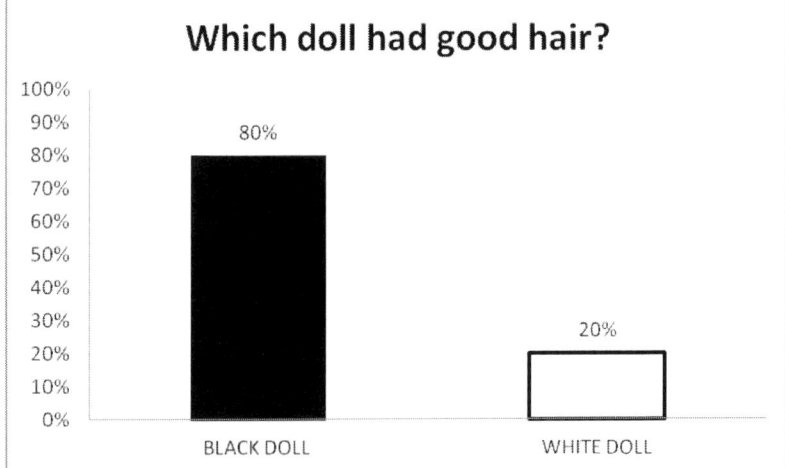

Which doll had good hair?

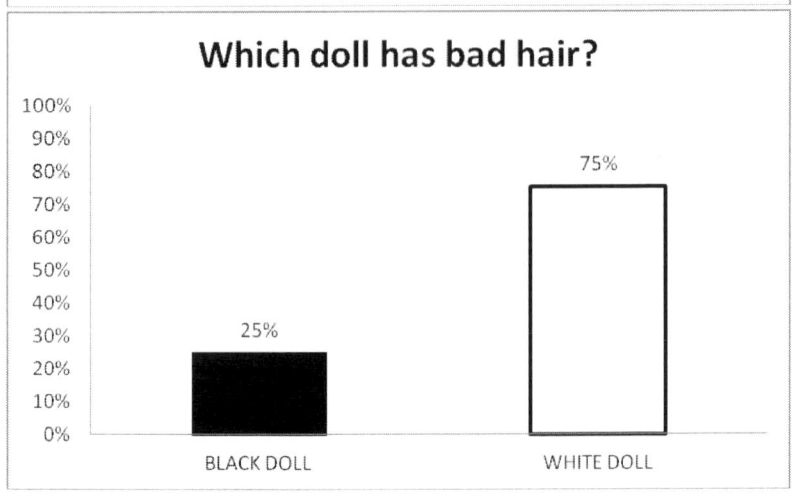

- BLACK DOLL: 80%
- WHITE DOLL: 20%

Which doll has bad hair?

- BLACK DOLL: 25%
- WHITE DOLL: 75%

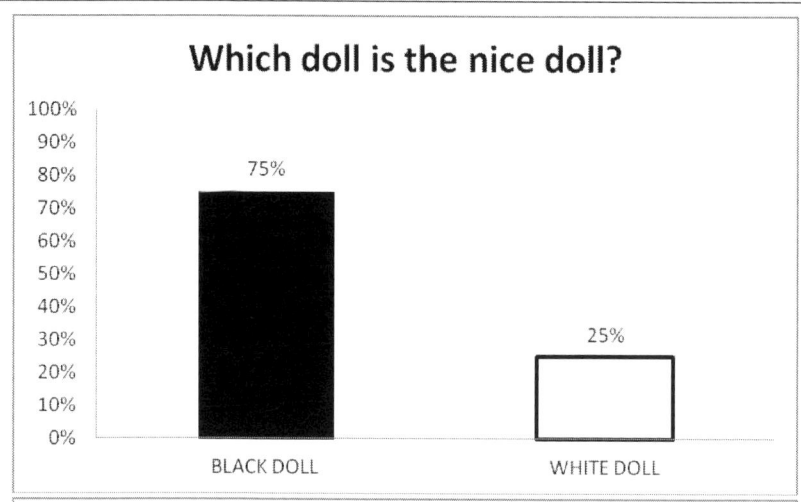

Kissi Kurls

Which doll is the nice doll?

- BLACK DOLL: 75%
- WHITE DOLL: 25%

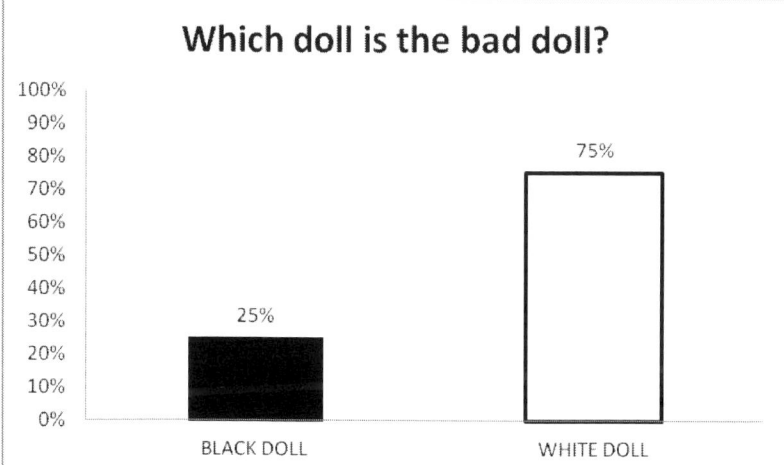

Which doll is the bad doll?

- BLACK DOLL: 25%
- WHITE DOLL: 75%

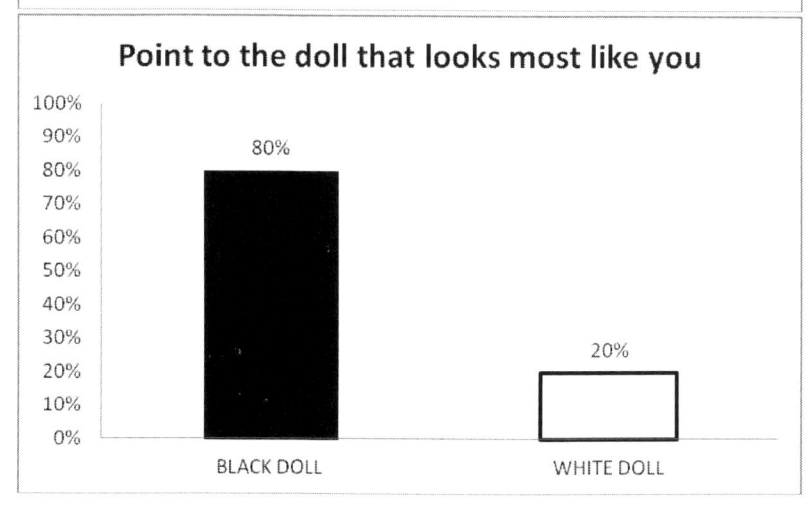

Point to the doll that looks most like you

- BLACK DOLL: 80%
- WHITE DOLL: 20%

www.KissiKurls.com

Conclusion of the Natural Hair Doll Experiment

Previous iterations of the doll test experiment showed that black children would routinely select the white doll as 'prettier, nicer', and having more positive qualities over the black doll. However, the Natural Hair doll test was carried out amongst a community of parents who had made a point of instilling self-confidence and love of natural hair within their children. An overwhelming majority of the children selected the Black doll to be prettier, nicer, and have more positive qualities over the white doll.

The Natural hair doll test was the first test in which the Black doll actually had a hair texture which was more like the Natural hair texture of Black people, and in the test the overwhelming majority of the children liked the Black doll over the White doll.

This experiment was conducted to promote positive identity amongst our black children. If children are nurtured to love self, then the self-loathing that exists within our community can be replaced with more positive images and self worth. The combination of parents teaching and instilling self-confidence and love of Natural hair, as well as having dolls which not only look like Black children, but also have hair textures like that of the natural hair texture of Black people, are ways to positively promote natural Black beauty standards amongst Black people.

*The experiment can be seen on www.youtube.com/user/kissikurls *Natural Hair Doll Test*.

Chapter Six

B.O.B- Black Owned Business

In order to survive and thrive we have to support Black Owned Businesses. When we support our own, we strengthen our economy, community, and relationships. I wanted to include this section in my book because I have noticed that there are a large number of Black Owned Businesses (B.O.Bs) especially within the cosmetic sector. There are more African inspired clothing outlets, accessories sources and natural product and service retailers than there used to be. This increase has transpired, I feel, due to the large numbers of women wanting to go natural and creating their own natural products, of which most of the ingredients can be easily sourced at the local, natural health stores and/or the kitchen cupboard. I want to emphasize the importance of supporting one another and sticking together, so that we are able to build a strong business foundation for future generations. The large number of black owned business has come about, in my opinion, due to a lack of provision: services, resources, etc., which are needed within our community. The natural hair movement has inspired many sistas & brothas too, to be self employed providing services geared towards our people for the benefit of our people. In relation to this, the phrase FUBU (For Us By Us) comes to mind. As a result we are creating more jobs in our communities and this is clearly great news!

I had a conversation with a friend of mine who owns a catering company. She told me that she was delighted to hear that her daughter, who spoke so confidently before, about working in a bank, now wants to own her own business, following in the footsteps of her parents. Images are so powerful, it's important that a child has good role models. This will help nurture them to be self-reliant, proactive individuals within the community. When I think of Black Wall Street, an affluent community of black owned business operating in 1921, it stirs up a lot of positive emotions for me. More importantly though, it encourages me to focus and strive for success, in all areas of my life.

The Top Ten Non-Black Owned Products/Services That Black Folk Think Are Black Owned

The services/ products listed below in a web article named 'The madman chronicles' have black faces on their brand however they are not black owned:

- Black Entertainment Television
- Def Jam Records
- Marc Ecko
- Jimmy Jazz
- Essence Magazine
- The Game
- The George Foreman Grill
- Church's Chicken
- Popeye's Chicken
- T.V. One
- SoftSheen Carson

"The black British entrepreneur, almost invisible in public consciousness, is more and more common in fact. A report by the Department of Trade and Industry shows that nearly half of black-owned businesses have been trading for less than three years, reflecting an upward trend, with more moving away from niche services such as black hairdressing and catering, and into the mainstream, especially the IT sector. There are 10,000 black-owned businesses in London, accounting for 4% of all firms in the capital and bringing in £4.5bn for the nation's coffers, with many thousands more across the country. And the numbers are growing.

The business savvy website Black Business Network reported that Black owned businesses in the United States increased 60.5% between 2002 and 2007 totaling of 1.9 million Black firms. From retail to restaurant industry African Americans are opening businesses and growing by epic leaps and bounds across America. Black owned businesses are currently grossing over 137 Billion per year. Here are some profiles of just a few such entrepreneurs from around the world, who may not otherwise get the media attention they deserve:

Clarence Otis Jr. - Darden

Darden is the world's largest full service restaurant operating company with annual sales of more than $8.5 billion. The company owns and operates more than 2,100 Red Lobster, Olive Garden, Longhorn Steakhouse, Bahama Breeze, Seasons 52, The Capital Grille, Eddie V's and Yard House restaurants in North America. Darden employs more than 200,000 people and serves more than 425 million meals annually. In 2013, Darden was named in FORTUNE's '100 Best Companies to Work For 'list, for the third year in a row.

Piers Linney, CEO of Outsourcery

Outsourcery is the UK's first carbon neutral Unified Communications and Hosted Information Technology Solutions Company. Piers, as CEO, also possess a broad breadth of professional experience, having qualified as a solicitor and worked as an investment banker, venture capital fund manager and hedge fund manager.

With a £44 million annual turnover, the Outsourcery venture catapulted Piers into becoming the UK's most successful black entrepreneur.

Aliko Dangote-The Dangote Group

The Dangote Group which started up as a small trading firm was established in 1977. Today, it is a multi-trillion naira conglomerate with many of its operations in Benin, Ghana, Nigeria, and Togo. At present, Dangote has enlarged his line of businesses to also cover food processing, cement manufacturing, and freight. A Nigerian business magnate with a net worth of $16.1 billion, he is the world's richest black person, according to Forbes magazine's 2013 ranking of the world's richest people.

Charles Orgbon III (2013) CEO and Founder of Greening Forward

Charles Orgbon III is a student at Mill Creek High School in Dacula, Georgia and the CEO and Founder of Greening Forward, an organization that establishes, engages and empowers a diverse global environmental movement powered by young people. At age 12, Orgbon noticed his school's littering problem and started a student club to take charge of school beautification projects. Orgbon and his peers integrated environmental education into the school curriculum, planted school gardens, started a composting program and led recycling initiatives. He now leads a team of 30 to help other young people be a part of the world's environmental solution.

Alex and Feysan Lodde-MV Transportation Inc

The Fairfield, California company, founded in 1975 by a husband-and-wife team, Alex and Feysan Lodde, has nearly 13,000 employees and revenue of more than $700 million annually. Its 7,000 vehicles serve public and private passengers in 100 locations in 26 states of the USA as well as Canada. The Fairfield, California company is the nation's 'largest privately held passenger-transportation contracting firm'.

Ulysses "Junior" Bridgeman -Bridgeman Foods Inc.

Ulysses "Junior" Bridgeman is owner and president of $500 million Manna Inc. and ERJ Inc. which manage more than 320 restaurants. These include 163 Wendy's Old Fashioned Hamburger restaurants, 120 Chili's, nine Perkin's Family Restaurants and Bakery restaurants and at least 28 Fazoli's.

Lonnie Johnson (inventor)

In 1980 Johnson formed his own law firm and licensed the Super Soaker water gun to Larami Corporation. Two years later the Super Soaker generated over $200 million in retail sales and became the best selling toy in America. Johnson reinvested a majority of his earnings from the Super Soaker into research and development for his energy technology companies - "It's who I am, it's what I do" He says. Currently, Johnson holds over 80 patents, with over 20 more pending, and is the author of several publications on spacecraft power systems.

The RLJ

Robert L Johnson and Thomas J. Baltimore Jr. co-founded and then acquired 22 properties worth more than $1 billion. They include two hotels in New York; five properties in the Washington, D.C. area and hotels in Tampa, Florida and Los Angeles. The firm's 2010 revenue was $578 million.

Janice Bryant Howroyd

Companies with staffing, human resources or business concerns consult Bryant Howroyd, who has built a firm generating nearly $1 billion in annual revenue. The North Carolina A&T University graduate founded ACT-1, headquartered in Torrance, California in 1978, and is CEO of what is now the nation's largest woman- and minority-owned employment-services company.

CAMAC International Corporation.

President Obama enlisted a seasoned entrepreneur when he appointed Kase Lawal to the Advisory Committee for Trade Policy and Negotiation. In 1986 the Nigerian-born chairman and CEO of CAMAC, founded his company, which has an annual revenue of about $1.5 billion, to explore, develop and operate oil properties. Lawal, who has a B.Sc. in chemical engineering and an MBA, worked as a chemist and a chemical engineer prior to starting CAMAC in Houston, Texas.

Just do it!

There is so much we can learn from Black Wall Street. It is fundamental that we, as a people, replicate this very model in order to gain a good standing in society, so that we will be in a position to command power and respect amongst one another and with our counterparts of other races.

I imagine life, back then was so much harder than it is now, and yet our community hasn't moved that much further forward. Although we may like to think that having an African American president somehow erases the reality of the state of our community, it does not, and cannot. We need to start at a local level and be consistent in order for there to be an impact. The change starts with us!

I made a conscious decision in 2008 to support B.O.B. Where better to make use of one's hard earned cash by putting it back into the community? What better an event than for a wedding! After all, collectively we have the 'buying power'. Black consumers spent, in 2009, an estimated $507 billion in 27 product and services categories…..exactly!

Across all communities it is estimated that 2.5 million brides get married each year. The wedding industry makes a fortune as some brides spend in excess of $16,000 for their wedding arrangements. With this in mind we decided that we would make a conscious effort to employ B.O.B for our wedding. I had four months to plan a 'destination' wedding, no dress no venue 'not a thing' prepared. I was on a mission to seek B.O.B to be a part of my special day. When I told friends and family what I intended to do everyone commended my efforts but many were concerned that it would be a tall order. I was determined, however, and I planned to succeed.

The process

When sourcing vendors, I would try and find out who owned the company by checking on the company website and doing a web search on their names. This would save me a lot of time, as in some cases where a website wasn't available; I would have to call the business.

In such cases I would find out, for example, when calling catering companies, who I felt understood the importance of having ones special cultural dish for such an occasion. After establishing a rapport and finding out what their specialties were, I would ask if it was a B.O.B. The majority were forth coming; a few clearly wanted my business, and although not B.O.B they tried to convince me that they were able to cook dishes such as Jollof rice and suchlike. Now, Jollof rice, when cooked correctly, will have your taste buds dancing so I wasn't going to take any chances. I found out that the majority of catering companies commonly served pasta and cold Hors d'œuvre and I wanted traditional African or Caribbean food. I guess that given hard times and it being a recession, naturally businesses will push for sale even if it costs them their integrity. However, I was intent on ensuring that this wedding was authentically B.O.B.

My list was uniformly being ticked off daily as I had sourced from the web and filtered out businesses that were not suitable. I had collated a list of B.O.B professionals, skilful and approachable, coupled with good customer services and reviews. Although two of the vendors were not B.O.B., one being the source of my wedding dress and the other being the venue, but which was a facility that helped children who suffered with sickle cell, learning disabilities and generally children in need. This latter facility assured me that 80% of the cost of the venue would go to the children in need, so I was ecstatic to say the least. Sometimes one has to weigh up the situation and see what makes sense, and to me that was a done deal.

A result! I received remarks like:
- "That was the best wedding I have ever been to!"
- "Where did you find all those vendors? It was amazing!"
- "Just beautiful!" that last remark was for me...hurrah!

A few people noticed that all the vendors were B.O.B. and so they were happy to be a part of my special day for more reasons than one. I had achieved my goal; demonstrating that it is possible to find within an industry such as the weddings one, hard-working, business-savvy, black professionals within the community. There is no doubt about it! If only you are willing to invest the time, and the effort, the results can be a win -win situation. As the saying goes a house divided cannot stand.

"The value of sourcing B.O.B professionals is the icing on the cake. Working together as a unit makes us an unstoppable force!"

Take action! Think. When you spend your money outside of your community, will the end user, the one that benefits from the transaction be someone that looks like you? Are you one of those people who say, 'I don't care!'? Well, my friend, that is the problem. Some of our people just do not care. There is a Caribbean proverb which says, 'Don't care was made to care!' Meaning that a lack of attention to the need to care will surely reveal itself to the non-carer.

The moment that we start caring about where we spend our money; the type of partner we choose; how the children are raised; the importance of excelling; then we will all see a positive change within our community. Our overall behavior and choices affect not just us but our community too, as they say among the Akan tribe 'We are all one'.

Make a conscious effort to spend your money predominately with B.O.Bs. You may decide to switch from large, commercially owned grocery stores to local farmers markets that are privately owned or decide that there is a niche and capitalize on the lack of B.O.B grocery stores yourself. Perhaps you can decide to buy cultural food from African or Caribbean outlets and get the toiletries from the commercial shop. However you decide, make a conscious choice to give back to the community, even if it's just one business you support, the key here is start and then continue to support!

Last year a friend of mine emailed me a link about a couple who decide to buy black products for a year. Maggie Anderson started "The Empowering Experiment" to see if she and her husband could patronize only black-owned businesses. It is an interesting insight into the determination and strength of the couple, who were determined to support black owned businesses.

The emotional highs and lows of their experiment are documented in a book entitled, 'Our Black Year' by Maggie Anderson. It is recommended reading!

Tips for sourcing pros

When sourcing for new business you want to be certain that they are legitimate, efficient and professional. Here are a few tips to ensure that you get a quality service.

Ask friends and family first for recommendations before, resorting to the internet, yellow pages or other agents.

Look at the company's history. Are they a genuine B.O.B? Who are the owners? How long have they been in business?

Check out customer reviews to give you a general feel. Remember not everything you read on the internet is true, so research widely, use your judgment, and research again.

Interview the potential vendor. After all, it is a job they are going to perform, so treat it as such.

Go to the place of business, where you can, see how they operate. Ensure that your values and theirs are compatible and that the person you are dealing with understands your wants and needs.

Are they a person of their word? If they say they are going to call, for example and they don't and this happens routinely, move on. This is inconsistency and when doing business this is a pitfall you'd want to avoid.

If they do a good job commend their services, everyone likes to be praised for things they are good at. So recommend and post a review, so that other people can benefit from such a service. Likewise, if your experience is the reverse, do let the company know your concerns in a poised and respectful manner. Shouting and insulting will not resolve anything, neither will it change anything. The approach matters, so tread carefully, and do post a review if the issues are not addressed in a timely manner so that others will not be at the mercy of such a business.

Having worked as a customer service manager, I know the importance of great customer service and the impact it can have on a business. Having repeat business is a goldmine that gives you steady income and happy loyal customers. This is what every business should strive for. However, unfortunately this basic simple rule within our community seems to fall on deaf ears. It baffles me as to why some people are employed in a customer service facing role, when they clearly do not care about customers or the services that they receive.

I am sure that many of my readers have a few stories to tell about bad customer services and, believe me; I wouldn't hesitate in letting people know about my customer services experiences good or bad. So, how much does bad customer services cost the industry every year? I was shocked but not surprised that by the below statistics:

- $289 is the average value of every lost business relationship in the U.S. per year
- 71% of consumers ended a business relationship due to a poor customer service experience
- 61% of customers take their business to a competitor after a poor customer service experience

- The estimated cost in United States of bad customer services to the financial industry is estimated 44 billion dollars a year!

It may seem like commonsense but, as they say, common sense is not always so common. To improve your retention of satisfied customers, treat them how you would like to be treated. Here are a few responses I have heard and experienced. These are some golden rules in order to keep happy and loyal customers.

He/she had a really bad attitude. So I left and won't be going back.

Place feedback cards in your business structure interface with the client. In this way you will become aware of the potential weaknesses within the business so that these can be identified and resolved. The right attitude is key. Your representatives are the face of your company therefore, it is vital that they uphold the company's rules, procedures and etiquette when interacting with customers. If the customer has left feedback with contact information, contact the customer and ask for more detailed feedback to retain their custom. Offer a goodwill gesture, the key is to make the customer feel valued.

The representative was not friendly and they were acting as if I was doing them a favor by shopping there.

Greet and meet customers with a smile. I know we all have the odd off-days, however, do not take it out on staff or customers. At the very least remain pleasant, and respectful. It is a two way relationship! The customer is willing to support your business in return for services/goods which in turn puts food on your table, without customers you have no business.

I was left hanging on the phone for ages/walked into the shop and there was no one there to help me.

There should always be someone on hand to answer the phones or to be present in the company during business hours. Answering machines, though serving a purpose, can be annoying. A Huge number of sales are lost from companies not answering the phones or not being available. Implement a rota where the phones are always manned by your staff. Emphasize the importance of having company presence. Remember a phone call or walk-in customer is a potential sale.

Elite Agenda

I was watching a documentary about the 'Elite Agenda' recently. The term 'Elite Agenda' is a individual or a group of people who have an agenda to remain in power by any means necessary. I was amazed and astonished to know the lengths that these people - I will refer to them as 'puppet masters - will go to, to deceive the masses.

One of the discussions was about integration. Integration had nothing to do with black and white people coming together to live in love and harmony, it was more about capitalism. By way of explanation: back then in the Wind rush era black people had no choice but to go to one another for resources and trade. We were 'outcasts' and so, as a result, we supported each other's businesses. The result of this was that the black community had a strong bond, a sense of self, wealth and economic power. The 'puppet masters' were aware of this and had to find a way to divide our loyalties by giving us 'choice'. Choice meant the ability to choose between buying from ourselves or buying from the growing consumerist buying outlets. This meant that the black pound/ dollar would not remain in the black community for the duration of time that it had. Ultimately this broke down our economic structure and power.

The same story can be applied to women's liberation. It had much less to do with equal rights for women and their having the same footing as men. It was much more about capitalism: enabling women to participate in the consumerist economy. This is how the capitalist, pro-growth economy thinks. They make you think that they are doing 'good', whilst their agenda has always been to benefit themselves. Think, if there are two people in the household and taxes are only being paid by one member of the household, how does one plan to get tax from the other member of the household, the woman, unless it is by defaming her role of a house wife and encouraging her to go to work which results in her now paying tax. The household has thus been converted into one in which now two people are paying tax.

This also results in her spending less time with the children, which negatively affects the mother and child bond. Children then become more at the mercy of the system. Teachers and other 'care-givers' are now raising our children, who are being referred to in some cases as delinquents. Black children who are inaccurately categorized as being difficult inevitably go on to be suspended from school and frustrated, because they are misunderstood. Children may then end up rebelling and end up in a child correction facility and, potentially, in a system of punitive relations. All of this as a result of the child not receiving the support and attention needed early on in its life-cycle.

With so many families caught up in the cycle of two working parents or single parenthood, it is now difficult to make meaningful interventions in the make-up of family structure. So, within this current system let's try to optimize our position by strengthening our community by patronizing our businesses. Let us reach out to our elders, neighbors, friends, and colleagues, and let us make these relationships work for us, affirmatively.

> *"**Being** good is commendable, but only when it is combined with **doing** good, is it useful."*

Product Junkie- Product Review

Product junkies, are you one of those? I will admit that I have accumulated a generous amount of hair products over the years. I was still searching for that one product that would actually do what it said on the package. Feeling disappointed that I could find a product that worked for my hair I decided to create KissiKurls. This product hydrates, nourishes moisturizes using natural ingredients. Some naturals enjoy product testing, however not the expense that comes with it. To maintain natural hair, all you really need is a great shampoo, conditioner, deep conditioner, moisturizer, oil, steamer, love and care. My advice is to support small B.O.B(Black owned Businesses) that have product lines with natural ingredients that are reasonably priced that will give you a more positive outcome for the health of your hair, Verses a grossly overpriced, highly publicized product that has harmful ingredients that could do more damage to your pocket, and the health of your hair. So if you are going to product test, then you need to accurately record your results. Below is a table that you can use to identify which products are agreeable or disagreeable for your hair.

Try and write down the results you obtain for each of the products you are using, so you can observe the effects of each and how your hair responds. A table has been created, for your convenience, for this purpose.

Kissi Kurls

Product	Does my hair feel dry? Y/N	Does my hair feel clean? Y/N	Does it feel soft? Y/N	Would I buy this again? Y/N	Observations	Rate 1-5 (1 disagreeable, 5 agreeable)

Love Your Natural Hair

Product	Does my hair feel dry? Y/N	Does my hair feel clean? Y/N	Does it feel soft? Y/N	Would I buy this again? Y/N	Observations	Rate 1-5 (1 disagreeable, 5 agreeable)

Hair Diary

<u>1 Year Anniversary</u>
How do I feel?

Love Your Natural Hair

My Healthy Hair Plan

1. My natural Hair Stylists name:
   Telephone Number:
   Address/Email:
   Website:

2. My natural Hair Stylists name:
   Telephone Number:
   Address/Email:
   Website:

What are my hair goals/plans?
_____
_____
_____
_____
_____
_____

1st Visit Hair Consultation
1._____
_____
_____

2._____
_____
_____

Plan of action:
1._____
_____
_____
_____

Love Your Natural Hair

2. _____

3. _____

4. _____

5. _____

6. _____

7. _____

Kissi Kurls

8. _____

9. _____

10. _____

11. _____

12. _____

Natural Hair Salons Directory

United Kingdom

London

Aquarius Hair Design
Sharon Parry
9 Stroud Green Road
Finsbury Park
London
N4 2DQ
Tel: 0207 263 2483

Junior Green
39 Knightsbridge
London, SW1X 7NL
Tel: 0207 752 0620

Locs Tafari Ltd
William Owusu/Daniel Okine
180a-182b Brownhill Rd
Catford
London
SE6 2DJ
Tel: 0208 695 0131
www.locstafari.com
info@locstafari.com

Back to Eden
Cynthia
20 Camberwell Road
Walworth Road
SE5 0EN
Tel: 0207 703 3173

KD Natural Hair
744 Holloway Road
London, Greater London
N19 3JF
Tel: 0207 263 0714

Morris Roots
Morris
21 Fulham High Street
London
SW6 3JH
Tel: 0207 731 7999
Tooting Brach: 184 Tooting High Street, London, SW17 0SF.
Tel: 020 8672 8003
www.morris-roots.com

Purely Natural
Anastasia
119 The Grove
Stratford, London
E15 1EN
Tel: 0208 221 0122
www.purelynaturalhair.com
Fb: Purely Natural Hair

The Hair Lounge
Charlotte Mensah
347 Portobello Road
London
W10 5SA
Tel: 0208 969 9444
www.hairlounge.co.uk
Fb: Portobello Hair Lounge

Tia's Hair Salon
72A Streatham HIll
London
SW2 4RD
Tel: 0208 623 9797
www.tiashairsalon.com
tia@tiashairsalon.com

Twist & Curves
Maria Thompson
www.twistcurves.com
Tel UK Salon: 07944 561 977
Tel USA Salon: 001 860 523 4844
Fb: Twist and curves

Toni and Guy - Covent Garden
Sabrina Natural Hair Stylist
4 Henrietta Street
Covent Garden
London
WC2E 8PS
Tel: 0207 240 7342

Manchester

Urban Sanctuary
110 Hulme High Street,
Manchester, Greater Manchester
M15 5JP
Tel: 01612 099583

Styles N Creations
Gege
Mobile Service
Manchester
Tel: 07506 630566

United States

Alabama

Hair Locks
Arlette
7000 E. Shea Blvd,
Ste. 1652 Scotsdale
AZ 85254
Tel: 480 443 7755

Irresistible Hair
Sonia Tutuwan Thames & Kelvin Thames
by appointment only
Birmingham, AL 35208
Tel: 205 529 0164/205 317 5767
www.irresistibleart.com

Locs of Soul
Tanene Jackson
3266 International Dr.
AL 36606
Tel: 240 515 4388
www.locsofsoul.com
curiosity4_u@yahoo.com

Natural Elements
1905 Bessemer Rd.
Birmingham, AL 35208
Tel: 205 788 2009
www.Naturalelementsbirmingham.com

Alaska

Totally Natural Hair Salon
1569 S. Bragaw St Suite 104
Anchorage, AK 99508
Tel: 907 338 8186
totallynatural4life@acsalaska.net

California

House of Venusian
Stewart
1608 Centinela St.
Suite 11
Inglewood, CA
Tel: 310 699 9788

Tangles & Locks
2025 Lake Ave.
Altadena, CA
Tel: (626) 398 9538

Margaret's Braids
1610 fulton Ave
Sacramento 95825
Tel: 916 203 9923
Margaretshairsalon.com
Margaretshairgaller@gmail.com

The Loc Loft
Aisha
by appointment only
Pomona, CA 91769
Tel: (909) 224 4152
www.thelocloft.com
thelocloft@gmail.com

Colorado

Hair Works
Tracey Moore
2201 Lafayette St,
Denver, CO 80205
Tel: 303 864 1585
Website: Hairworks@denver.com
Email: morehairworks@yahoo.com

Rumors Beauty Salon & Barber Shop
Precious Czeczok
14044 east Mississippi Avenue
Aurora, CO 80012
Tel: 502 819 6707/ 720 748 1400
www.Rumourshairsalons.com
Rumorshairsalons@gmail.com

It's Natural Hair Salon
Tayler Barber
299 Detroit St., Suite 109
Denver, CO 80247
Tel: 303 333 0219/ 720 641 7632
itsnatural2@gmail.com

Love Your Natural Hair

Connecticut

Baswa Hair Cultivating Studio
Brenda
65 Platt St #2
Hartford, CT 06103
Tel: 860 987 9707

Beloved Natural Hair Salon
Tayna Faucette Brooks
248 Farmington Ave
2nd Floor suite #209
Hartford, Connecticut
CT 06105
Tel: 860 794 2765
Belovedhair72@yahoo.com

Florida

A Nu Twist Multicultural Salon
813 W. University Avenue
Gainesville, FL 32601
Antoinette Black
Tel: 352 373 3300
flantblack@gmail.com

All Dolled Up Salons and Stores
Bailey
3453 N University Dr
Sunrise, FL 33351
Tel: 954 572 3336
sbaileyjr@adustyle.com

Black Star Unisex Salon
Forrest
1270D NW 31st Ave.
Ft. Lauderdale, FL 33311
Tel: 954 316 0036
www.blackstarworld.net

Coconuts Salon and Barber Shop
David
3366 NW 13th Street
Gainesville, FL 32609
Tel: 352 373 7323
davidblessedone@aol.com

Eloctricity Natural Hair Studio
Talvia Vereen
1011 NW 195th St.
Miami, FL 33169
Tel: 754 422 7970
www.facebook.com/HairbyTalvia
Eloctricity@gmail.com

Ethnic Hair Care
Tina
210 S. Kings Ave.
Suite P
Brandon, FL 33510
Tel: 813 643 5317
ethnichaircaresalon@gmail.com

Hair By Ned Jetti
Email: hair@nedjetti.com
Tel: 973 748 0181
www.hairbynedjetti.com

Mane Tain Natural Hair & Skin Care
Chana Darby
93 NE 125 St.
North Miami, FL 33161
Tel: 305 458 6635
manetainnatural@gmail.com

The Ebene Natural Hair Experience at Myra and Company
Erica
7313 Southwest 59th Court
Miami, FL 33143
Tel: 305 661 2381/ 305 234 1797
Website: miamispa.com

Lockstar Natural Retail & Salon
April Atkinson
1110 Morning Side Drive
Charlotte North Carolina 28205
Tel: 704 737 4455
April Atkinson.com
Fb: April Atkinson
info@lockstar.com

Natural Trend Setters
Simone Hylton & Yanique Hylton
7247 Nw 88th Avenue
Tamarac Florida 33321
Tel: 954 486 1414
Fb: Natural Trend Setters
www.natualtrendsetters.com

Tru Roots
David Daniel
Jacksonville, FL
Tel: 904 389 0848
truroots@earthlink.net

Georgia

All Creations Salon
976 Main St
Stone Mountain, GA 30083

Best Braids
Angela Davis
1164 Clark Ave
Albany, GA 31705
Tel: 229 878-0778

Bangz & Tanglez
2617 Panola Road, STE 104
Lithonia, Georgia 30038
Tel: 770 322-0322

Debby's Hair Braiding
Tel: 770 712 0258
Info@debbyhairbraiding.com
www.debbyhairbraiding.com

Deeply Rooted
2443 Spring Rd SE,
Smyrna, GA 30080
Tel: 770 436-2400
info@deeplyrootedhair.com
www.deeplyrooted.com

Lifestyle Of The Rich & Kinky
Yarrow
3480 Greenbriar Parkway
Atlanta Suite 126
GA 30331
Tel: 404 221 8900
Yarrow7777@gmail.com
www.richandkinky.com

Natural Xpressions Salon
383c Marietta St corner
suite (2nd floor)
Atlanta
GA 30313
Tel: 404 856 0641
www.naturalxpressionsalon.com

Salon International
Maureen Rowe
1070 Mistletoe Road
Decatur Georgia 30033
Styles707@gmail.com
Tel: 443 220 3064

The Nappy Parlour
Tara Davis
nappyparlor@bellsouth.ne
Tel: 404 755 4626

Hawaii

Braids Hawaii
Sandy
1415 Kalakaua Ave. Ste. 216
Honolulu, HI 96826
Tel: 808 951-9700
www.braidshawaii.com

Illionis

Chatto
65 E. Oak St.
Chicago, IL 60611
www.chattoecofriendlysalon.com
Tel: 312 640 0003

Desi's Full Salon Service salon
2130 West 95th Street
Chicago
Il 60643
Tel: 773 445 8300
Email: nywele@ymail.com

Twisted Roots Salon
701 East 75th Street
Chicago 60619
Tel: 773 895 4968
Twistedrootssalonin@yahoo.com
www.twistedrootssalon.vpweb.com

Daryas Natural Hair Boutique
2134 S Michigan
Chigago Il 60616
Tel: 312 225 7620
www.daryanaturalhaircare.com

Naturally U Hair Salon
Kim Willis MBA
4875 W. 56th St Suite E
Indianapolis, IN 46254
317 295-8905
www.minenaturally.net

Kansas

KC Styles
4301 State Avenue
Kansas City, KS 66102
Tel: 347-404-4070

Styles Of Essence Salon
5908 Woodson
Mission Kansas
66202
Tel: 816 694 6514
www.StylesofEssenceHair.com
Sherheafrazier@comcast.net

Louisiana

Tru Rootz Natural Hair Salon
Cornell
3351 Kabel Drive
Ste D
New Orleans, LA 70131
Tel: 504-433-8198
Truroots@yahoo.com

Maryland

Dreadz N' Headz
1826 Woodlawn Dr.
Woodlawn, MD 21207
Tel: 410-298-0660
www.dreadznheadz.com
ohnappy1@aol.com

Holistic Hair Care
Ansylla's
8604 Central Ave, Suite 4
Landover, MD 20785
Tel: 301 328-2941 Voicemail

Urban Nature Natural Haircare
1903 Seminary Road
Silver Spring, MD
Tel: 301-747-9090
www.urbannaturestyles.com
info@urbannaturestyles.com

Michigan

Happy To Be Nappy
Tel: 313 340 4247
www.happytobenappysalon.com

4 Our Daughters
Wendy
Tel: 734 252 6511
4ourdaughtersinc@gmail.com

Missouri

Into Hair Naturally
Teresa Miller
7601 Troost Avenue
Kansas city
Missouri
64131
Tel: 816 523 0073
www.n2hairnaturally.com

Naturally Trendy Natural Hair
Kinshasa
5921A Troost Avenue Suite A
Kansas City, Missouri 64110
Tel: 816 214 8899
www.Naturallytrendysalon.com
naturallytrendy@gmail.com
Fb Naturally Trendy Natural Hair

Your Natural Image
645 E 59th Street
Kansas City Missouri 64110
Tel: 816 444 4048
www.Shaun@YourNaturalImage.com
Your naturalimage.com
Fb Your Natural Image

New Jersey

Meko
616 Freeman Street
Orange NJ 07111
Tel: 862 438-8630
info@mekonewyork.com

New Mexico

Kamaria Creations Natural Hair and Skin Care Center
1501 Mountain Rd NW
Albuquerque, NM 87104
Tel: 505-244-9104
www.kamariacreations.com/
kamariacreations@aol.com

Natural Hair Designs
Melanie Kirven
Tel: 505-261-1746
www.Naturalhairdesigns.com
Melaniekirven@gmail.com

New York

H2 Salon
Dailey Greene
473 Tompkins Avenue
Brooklyn New York
NY 11216
Tel: 718 230-4225
www.h2bk.com

Locks & Chops
365 West 34Th Street #2,
New York, NY 10001
Tel: 212 244-2306
www.locksandchopsnyc.com

Hair rules salon
828 9th avenue,
(between 54th & 55th streets)
suite one
New York, 10019
Tel: 212.315.2929
www.hairrulessalon.com

Natural Hair Salon in Brooklyn
663 Nostrand ave
Between St Marks and Prospect Pl
Brooklyn, NY 11216
Tel: 718 484-7833
www.bohemiansoul.com
appt@bohemiansoul.com

Ohio

Natures Outer Beauty Salon
Sarah
5254 Section Ave
Cincinnati, OH 45212
Tel: 513-351-7111
www.naturesouterbeautysalon.com

Stephano & Co & Reverence Design Team
Zakke Ali Natural Hair Stylist
Tel: 216 921 4242

Tennessee

Naturally You Salon
3926 Gallatin Pike Suite C
Nashville
Tennessee
37216
Tel: 615 485 6936
www.naturallyyousalon.com

Natural Awakenings Hair Salon
7009 Lennox Village Drive Suite 104
Nashville Tennessee 37211
Tel: 615 669 1563
naturalawakenings123@gmail.com
www.vagaro.com/NaturalAwakenings

Washington D.C.

Cornrows & Company
Pamela Ferrell
5401 14th St., NW
Washington, DC 20011
Tel: 202 723 1827
talknhair@cornrowsandco.com

Twist It Sistah
Adjuana Crawford
317 T St., NE
Washington, DC 20002
Tel: 202 832 3157
Email: adjuanacrawford@gmail.com

Urban Nature
2802 Georgia Ave., NW
Washington, DC 20001
Tel: 202 332 2001
info@urbannaturestyles.com

Disclaimer
The purpose of this directory is to provide a Resource which lists hair salons, the author disclaims all liability, and individual accepts full responsibility and liability on their decision whether or not they choose to patronize these establishments.

Credits

Books:

1. Develop Your Inner Beauty. "The Secret" by Rhonda Byrne

2. Do you Lye? 'Toxic Beauty 'How Hidden Chemicals in Cosmetics Harms You'. Dawn Mellowship

3. Hair Facts - 'The complete Royal families Of Ancient Egypt' Aiddan Dodson & Dyan Hilton

4. Hair facts - 'The civilization of Ancient Egypt.' Paul Johnson

5. Hair Tips 'Living Beauty' -Bobbi Brown

6. Hair Tips, Healthy Eating 'Cosmetics Unmasked Level 1' Dr Stephen & Gina Antczak

7. Hair Tips 'Introducing Hairdressing' Christine Mcmillian-Bodell

8. Hair Tips 'Beauty Therapy 2nd Edition Level 2 ' Jane Hiscock & Frances Lovett

9. Hair Tips 'Hairdressing 3rd Edition' Bob Woodhouse

10. Hair Type Hype? - 'Supreme Mathematic African Maat Magic'- African Creation Energy

11. Healthy Eating, Hair Tips' Beauty Therapy fact file 4th Edition' Susan Cressy

12. Interesting Hair Facts - 'Reader Digest Journey into the past. Life in the land of the Pharaohs'

13. Mirror Mirror On The Wall - "Theory and Practice of Counseling and Psychotherapy" sixth edition, by Gerald Corey

14. The Good, The Bad & Ugly Ingredients - 'Don't Go to the cosmetic counter without me' 7th edition author Paula Begoun

15. The Good, The Bad, & Ugly Ingredients - 'The Rough Guide To Ethical Living' Duncan Clark

Photo Credits:
1. Do You Lye? Serena Williams- celebrityhairloss.blogspot.com/2011/10/are-hair-extensions-to-blame-for-serena.html

2. Do You Lye? Oprah Winfrey huffingtonpost.com/2009/04/24/oprah-defends-her-hair-th_n_191287.html

3. Hair Facts -bglhonline.com/wp-content/uploads/2011/04/africanhair.jpg

4. Hair Facts- historylink101.net/egypt_1/a-hair_styles.htm

5. Hair Facts -egyptsearch.com/forums/ultimatebb.cgi?ubb=print_topic;f=15;t=004214

6. Hair Facts-Photos taken by Dinah Kissiedu

7. Hair Gallery-Photos taken by Dinah Kissiedu

8. Hair Storeis - President Barack Obama Bending down. Iowntheworld.com

9. Hair Type Hype-The Number, Nine- numerology.com

10. Rocking your fro on the go-Model-Threading source: www.thenaturalhavenbloom.com

Journals:
1. Do You Lye? -Hair European Journal of Dermatology (14:1, pp28-32, 2004)

2. Do You Lye? - American Journal o f Epidemiology-chemical hair treatments & adverse pregnancy among black women in central north Carolina AMJ Epidemol Vol 149 No.8 1999

3. Do You Lye? American Journal of Epidemiology 2012;175(5):432-40. doi: 10.1093/aje/kwr351. PMCID: PMC3282879.

4. Hair Facts - American Journal o f Epidemiology. (2012) Wise LA, Palmer JR, Cozier YC, Rosenberg L. Hair relaxer use and risk of uterine leiomyomata in African American women.

5. Hair Structure-dralisyed.com/hairdamage Cuticles-Dr N Syed President & Master Chemist

Internet Credits:

1. Black Owned Business - http://blackdemographics.com/economics/black-owned-businesses

2. Black Owned Business- Bartering system - money.howstuffworks.com/bartering.htm

3. Black Owned Business- www.blackbusinessnetwork.com

4. Black Owned Business-blog.kissmetrics.com/customer-service

5. Black Owned Business-www.forbes.com

6. Black Owned Business -www.theroot.com

7. Black Owned Business -sfbayview.com/2011/what-happened-to-black-wall-street-on-june-1-1921 – black wall street

8. Do You Lye? - toxnet.nlm.nih.gov/cgi-bin/sis/search/a?dbs+hsdb:@term+@DOCNO+7167

9. Do You Lye? Oprah - http://www.huffingtonpost.com/2009/04/24/oprah-defends-her-hair-th_n_191287.html

10. Essential Oils-skinbiology.com/truthabouthairrelaxers.html

Kissi Kurls

11. Hair Colour-livestrong.com/article/69199-demi-permanent-vs.-semi-permanent/

12. Hair Dead or Alive- wikipedia.org/wiki/Hair

13. Hair Dead or Alive-christiannature.blogspot.com/2009/08/help-your-plants-talk-to-them-and-play.html

14. Hair Dead or Alive?-rps.psu.edu/probing/talkingtoplants.htm

15. Hair Dead or Alive?-livestrong.com/article/395065-what-vitamins-minerals-promote-hair-regrowth/

16. Hair Facts-ukhairdressers.com/history%20of%20hair.asp

17. Hair Facts-topix.com/forum/afam/TVN2F06ECU7PRF2O4

18. Hair Facts-raceandhistory.com/historicalviews/ancientamerica.htm

19. Hair Facts-thenaturalhaven.blogspot.com/2010/08/does-male-hair-grow-faster-than-female.html

20. Hair Facts-walterporterhair.com/component/content/article/50-did-you-know/76-the-removal-of-unwanted-body-hair-can-be-dated-back-to-the-time-of-the-ancient-egyptians

21. Hair Loss - alopeciaonline.org.uk/types-of-alopecia.asp

22. Hair Loss-Alopecia- aarda.org/patient_information.php

23. Hair Loss -blackhealthzone.com/black-women-and-hair-loss

24. Hair Stories-Rhonda Lee-www.huffingtonpost.com

25. Hair Tips -hair-heads.co.uk/hair-colour/permanent-hair-colour.php

26. Hair Tips-naturalblackhaircare.com/waystogrowhair.php

27. Hair Tips-vivawoman.net/2008/08/08/is-it-better-to-wash-our-hair-in-cold-water/

28. Healthy Eating-suite101.com/article/vitamins-for-hair-growth-a60366

29. Inner Beauty-Elders -unity4power.org/eldercouncil.html

30. Interesting Hair Facts-gurmat.info/sms/smspublications/thesikhsymbols/chapter7/

31. Rocking Your Natural Fro Photos-Hair Styles - naturalbeautifulhair.com

32. The Good, The Bad, & Ugly Ingredients -preventcancer.com

33. The Good, The Bad, & Ugly Ingredients-osha.gov Occupational Safety & Health Organization

34. The Good, The Bad, & Ugly Ingredients -LUKAS, S. E.. "Rubbing Alcohol." Encyclopedia of Drugs, Alcohol, and Addictive Behavior. 2001. Retrieved November 08, 2012 from Encyclopedia.com:

35. The Good, The Bad, & Ugly Ingredients- Csaky, T. Z., & Barnes, B. A. (1984). Cutting's handbook of pharmacology, 7th ed. Norwalk, CT: Appleton-Century-Crofts.

36. The Good, The Bad & Ugly Ingredients - American Journal Of contact Dermatist, September 2000, 165-169 and Acta Demato Venerelogical November 1999 pages 418-421

37. The Good, The Bad, & Ugly Ingredients- AloeSajten.com

38. The Good, The Bad, & Ugly Ingredients-humanesociety.org/issues/cosmetic_testing/

39. Transitioning Or Big Chop- Aaron McGruder creator of the Boondocks in Afro Denial and Ethono-ambiguo Hostility-The Real Afrikan Truth

Illustration:
- African Creation Energy
- Santiago

Hair Models:
- Chantel Smith
- Evone Hinds-Hair By Vin Kiss Kat
- Natural Lounge Event in London -Hair Gallery
- Rocking Your Fro Models: Locks, Blowout, Bantu, Threading, Natural Beautiful Hair.com
- Yonkel Chamberlain

Makeup Artist/Hair Stylist:
- Bangz & Tanglez Hair Salon, Felecia Golden-Jones
- Visage "Faces" by Naomi
- Yonkel Chamberlain

Photographers:
- Dinah Kissiedu
- Kevin Goolsby
- Yonkel Chamberlain

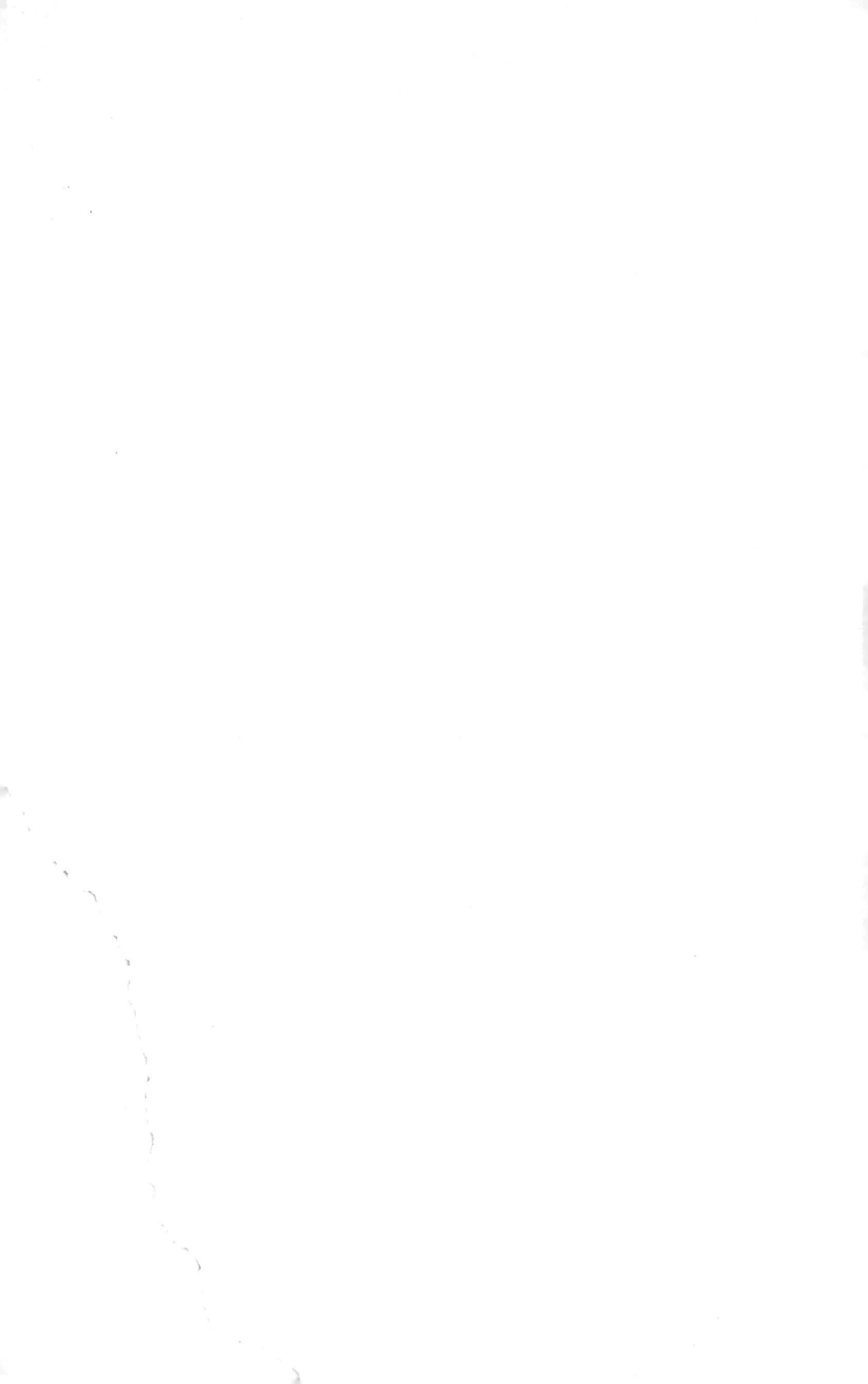